DISABILITY
AND
ORAL CARE

EDITED BY
DR JUNE NUNN

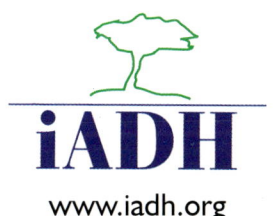

iADH

www.iadh.org

ISBN 0 9539261 0 9

Published by FDI World Dental Press Ltd
7 Carlisle Street
London W1V 5RG, UK

Printed in Great Britain by Dennis Barber Graphics & Print, Lowestoft, Suffolk

Contents

Contributors

Bitte Ahlborg D.D.S.
Senior Consultant in Hospital Dentistry, Mun-H-Center, National Orofacial Resource Centre for Rare Disorders, Gothenburg, Sweden. Lecturer in dentistry and oral care services for persons with disabilities. Responsible for orofacial aids in the National Resource Centre. President of Nordic Association for Disability and Oral Health. Council member, International Association for Disability and Oral Health.

Jan Andersson-Norinder D.D.S
Senior Consultant in Hospital Dentistry, Director, Mun-H-Center, the National Orofacial Resource Centre for Rare Disorders in Gothenburg, Sweden. Secretary/Treasurer of the International Association for Disability and Oral Health.

Elinor Bouvy-Berends D.D.S
Senior Consultant in Special Care Dentistry; Director, Patient Care, Stichting Bijter, Centre for Special Care Dentistry, Rotterdam, The Netherlands. Past-President, Dutch Association for Dentistry for the Handicapped; council member, International Association for Disability and Oral Health. President, European Federation for the Advancement of Sedation and Anaesthesia in Dentistry (EFAAD). Lecturer in continuing postgraduate education courses on inhalation sedation and general anaesthesia.

Gary Enever MA (Cantab), MB BS (London) FRCA
Consultant anaesthetist with sessions at the Dental Hospital, Newcastle Hospitals NHS Trust. Clinical lecturer in Anaesthesia, University of Newcastle upon Tyne, England. His interests include audit, medical education (information technology) and history. Database coordinator, 'Current Opinions in Anaesthesiology'.

Janice Fiske BDS, FDS RCS Eng, Mphil
Senior lecturer / honorary consultant in Special Care Dentistry at Guy's, King's and St Thomas' Dental Institute of King's College London, England. Past President of the British Society of Gerodontology and the British Society for Disability and Oral Health. Honorary secretary for the British Society for Disability and Oral Health

Clive Friedman BDS Cert Ped Dentistry
Associate Clinical Professor, University of Western Ontario Department of Paediatric Dentistry, London, Ontario, Canada. Director Adult Disabilities Clinic, London Health Sciences Centre, London, Ontario, Canada. Past President, Academy of Dentistry for Persons with Disabilities (ADPD) and member of the Executive Committee of the International Association for Disability and Oral Health.

Janet Griffiths, LDS, BA(OU)
Associate Specialist/Special Care, Department of Adult Dental Health, University Dental Hospital, Cardiff, Wales, UK. Honorary Clinical Tutor. Past President of the British Society for Disability and Oral Health. Experience of General Dental Practice, Community Dental Service and Hospital Dental Service. Member of All Wales Special Interest Group - Special Care.

Daniel Jolly, DDS, FACD, FAAHD
Professor of Clinical Dentistry, Director, General Practice Residency. The Ohio State University College of Dentistry, Columbus, Ohio USA. Full time teaching, practice (and some research) in the area of special patient care for people with disabilities, severe medical problems and geriatric patients. Past President, IADH . Editor, IADH Journal. Secretary, Vice-President, American Association of Hospital Dentists.

Jenny King, BDS, PhD Dip Theol
Has extensive clinical experience as a dentist treating children and adults with special needs. She now teaches applied ethics and law to dental students at St Bartholomew's and the Royal London School of Medicine and Dentistry in East London, UK. Her current research is into consent in dental care.

Peter King, BDS MDS (Univ. of Sydney)
Staff specialist in special care dentistry at Westmead Hospital Dental Clinical School and clinical lecturer for the University of Sydney, Australia. He directs a unit that employs five FTE dental officers providing oral health care services for people with disabilities in New South Wales. Chairman of a steering committee to establish the Australian Society of Special Care in Dentistry.

Gunilla Klingberg, DDS, PhD
Senior consultant, Mun-H-Center, National Orofacial Resource Center for Rare Disorders, Göteborg, Sweden. Specialist degree in paediatric dentistry. Research focusing on psychological/behavioural spects of dental care, foremost dental fear/anxiety

Debbie Lewis, BDS, MPhil, MCCD RCS, Dip D Sed
Senior dental officer, Dorset Healthcare Community Dental Service, England. Developing and providing oral care services for adults with disabilities and people needing special care. Honorary Secretary for the British Society of Gerodontology. President-Elect for the British Society for Disability and Oral Health.

Graham Manley, BDS DDPH (RCS) MSc PhD
Senior Dental Officer-Special Needs, East Kent Community Dental Service, Engalnd. Regional Adviser in Community Dentistry for the Thames Region. Honorary Lecturer in Sedation and Special Care Dentistry at Guy's, King's and St Thomas' Dental Institute, London, England.

Paula Moynihan, BSc, SRD, PhD, RPHNutr. FRSA
Lecturer in Nutrition, School of Dentistry, University of Newcastle upon Tyne UK. Course leader for BDS course in Nutrition and Diet. Research interests include the cariogenic potential of glucose polymers and nutritional supplements and the diets of children with juvenile arthritis. President-Elect of the Nutrition Group of the International Association for Dental Research

June Nunn, BDS, DDPH, PhD, FDSRCS.
Senior Lecturer/Honorary Consultant in Paediatric Dentistry, School of Dentistry, University of Newcastle upon Tyne, UK. Degree Programme Director for the MSc in Disability and Oral Care at the University of Newcastle; Past President of both the British and International Association for Disability and Oral Health.

Lotta Sjögreen, BS
Speech therapist Mun-H-Center, the National Orofacial Resource Center for Rare Disorders in Göteborg, Sweden. Specialised in oral motor function and paediatric dysphagia.

Meg Skelly, MDS, FDSRCPS, FDSRCS.
Senior Lecturer & Consultant in Dental Sedation. Head of the Division of Community Dentistry, Sedation & Special Care Dentistry at Guy's, King's and St Thomas' Dental Institute, London, England. President of the Association of Dental Anaesthetists.

Kari Storhaug, DDS, Ph.D
Head of Department, Resource Centre for Oral Health in Rare Medical. Conditions, Dental Faculty, University of Oslo, Norway. Past President and Honorary Member of Nordic Society for Disability and Oral Health. President of the International Association for Disability and Oral Health.

Nick Watson, BSc (hons) MSc
Lecturer in the Department of Nursing Studies, University of Edinburgh, Scotland. He has published widely on disability related issues and his current research interests include work with disabled children. He is active in the disabled people's movement and is convenor of AccessAbility Lothian, Scotland.

Foreword

Lifelong learning is the commitment we make when we enter the caring professions. As part of its responsibility for education in the field of oral health care for people with disabilities, the International Association for Disability and Oral Health (IADH) has commissioned this textbook to help both undergraduate students and interested professionals, in their learning. The textbook brings together informed and experienced authors who detail the essential elements of their area of expertise. The views expressed therefore are those of the authors and do not necessarily represent IADH policy.

This book is dedicated to the memory of Marcel van Grunsven, a past president of IADH who died prematurely in February 1997. The concept of a textbook on oral care and disability belonged to Marcel. I would like also to acknowledge the contribution made by Dr Nobu Sakai and his Working Group on Quality Assurance. Much of what is contained within the document produced by this Group has provided the foundation for a number of the chapters in this textbook.

We are indebted to, principally, Colgate Palmolive and Unilever Dental Research, but also to The Dentists Provident Society and Cordent Dental Trust, for their support, without whom this venture would not have been possible.

June Nunn
Editor
Newcastle upon Tyne
July 2000

Chapter 1

Disability – a Context

June Nunn

Definitions

The whole ethos of this book surrounds the issue of reducing the disability imposed on people with impairments. Immediately however we are confronted by the semantics that surround definitions of disability.

Many people are familiar with the original ICIDH classification[1], which defined:

- Impairment as any loss or abnormality of physiological or anatomical structure or function,
- Disability is any restriction or lack (resulting from an impairment) of ability to perform an activity in a manner or within the range considered normal for a human being.
- Handicap is seen as the disadvantage for a given individual, resulting from an impairment or a disability, which limits or prevents the fulfilment of a role that is normal (depending on age, sex, social and cultural factors) for that individual.

Within the context of these definitions, there is little consensus as to what constitutes normality. This medical model attempts to link the experience of disabled people with that of the professionals treating them, that is, the patient must obey the professional in order to become well again.

The revised draft of the ICIDH[2] seeks to move away from this medical model to a bio-psycho-social model in order to encompass human function at the bodily, personal and social level. It will aim to remove the negative associations with handicap and replace it with the term 'participation'. The term 'disability' will be replaced by 'activity limitation'. The only dissent to this move away from the term 'handicap' is that in the past, this label has enabled people to obtain funding and services for which they would otherwise not have been eligible.

Thus, rather than attaching a label to someone as disabled we should be asking what is the person disabled for, not, what is their disability. Vygotsky[3] proposes identifying a person's strengths, rather than characterising the person as the sum of their negative characteristics. Crucial to the social model is the notion that activity limitation or the restriction in participation experienced has more to do with an unaccomodating environment, than to the individual's impairment. What is also becoming apparent is that the person is the primary consideration, not the defect; that is, the phrase is now 'people with disability' not disabled persons, or worse still, 'the disabled'[4].

Another issue in relation to definitions is that disability is not a dichotomous variable but rather a continuous one: renal failure exists as a degree and yet the decision to transplant a kidney is a yes/no decision. That is, treatment decisions are dichotomised[5]. Professionals like there to be neatness about the outcome; the search is always for a neat definition, on which to make recommendations. Kirchner[6] likens this to a drunken man looking for a coin under a lamppost instead of in the gutter where he dropped it. When asked why, he retorts that there was more light under the lamppost.

However, in United States law, if a person is registered as disabled, the more significant the disability the greater the protection against discrimination. So a continuum is permissible. Similarly, since the enactment of the 1995 English Disability Discrimination Act in 1999[7], those providing services for people with impairments are required to make reasonable attempts to accommodate those people with disabilities. In Canada, in 1995, the Quebec Professional Corporation of Dentists adopted an amendment to its Code of Ethics stating that a dentist cannot refuse to treat a patient for reasons related to the specific nature of a disease that a patient has nor for moral, political or language reasons. The dentist can however, if they judge it is in the best interests of the patient, refer the individual to another dentist.

Cultural variation

Much of what has gone before is new and will take time to permeate the culture of the western world. For some cultures the terminology will be entirely new. In African languages for example, there is no equivalent for 'handicap'. Rather there are words to describe observable impairments like lameness but no all- encompassing generic term.

Some cultures see names as stigmatising; in the United States mental retardation is an acceptable and currently used term whereas in other English-speaking countries outside the US this term has negative connotations.

Cultural differences impinge on people's approach to caring for relatives with impairments; Afro-Caribbean families are more inclined to rely on friends and inter-generational support than place relatives in long-stay institutions, despite poorer standards of living but perhaps because of larger families. Hispanic families too tend to look after relatives with disabilites believing it is a religious duty, a test by God of one's worthiness [8,9].

Ethics

Ethical dilemmas are ever present in clinical sciences. Genetic diseases and malformations are a major cause of disability and the potential to diagnose many defects ante-natally is now a reality. However, results from amniocentesis are not available until well into the second trimester when pregnancy is obvious. Tests that can be carried out earlier such as chorion villus sampling carry a higher risk of miscarriage. In order to make informed choices parents need to know how accurate the medical predictions are. Possessing this knowledge does not remove the trauma for prospective parents rather it enhances it in many cases. Some families have a deep-seated and irrevocable belief in the sanctity of life – a process that is continuous since the ovum is a living cell and fertilisation is only the process that brings about a mixing of genes. Imbuing the foetus with a persona at that stage may be premature since most of this early collection of cells is destined to become the placenta. Indeed, attributing a soul to this potential person begs the question of what happens when twins are conceived; is there a sharing of souls?

Families for whom the prospect of bearing a child with a disability have to tussle with difficult decisions made no easier by the relative primitiveness of the development of diagnostic tests. Parents often have high expectations of genetic counselling after the birth of a child with impairments and face disappointment when professionals are unable to clearly identify the origins of their child's defects. Parents may misinterpret a genuine lack of information as a conspiracy amongst health professionals to keep information from them or even not appreciating the seriousness of the situation that they, the parents, face[10].

Factors affecting the uptake of genetic counselling:

- perceived susceptibility to the condition(s)
- seriousness of the risk to health
- prospects for effective treatment
- plans to extend the family
- personal values and belief – especially as they relate to termination
- influence of other family members – with the condition
- gender
- possible loss of health insurance benefits

The objective view might be that it is in the best interest of parents and child if a foetus with a lethal impairment is aborted. This ignores the considerable guilt associated with the decision-making process and in this instance, allowing a natural conclusion which gives the parents a chance to grieve and come to terms with their loss, may be the preferred outcome (*Table 1*).

Clinicians are guided by the Hippocratic oath which states that they

Table 1. Rate per 1000 for inherited defects

Of notional 1000 pregnancies:	Prevalence	Hereditary defect
Miscarriages	150	1:2
Perinatal death	13	1:4
Severe retardation	16	3:4
Moderate retardation	38	3:4
Non-retarded	783	1:80

must do no harm: neonatologists can predict much from the condition of a baby and evidence from scans gives clues to the likely brain damage but some of the other medical complications cannot always be anticipated. Once the special care baby unit has embarked on a process of rescue, it can be difficult to know when to consider the withdrawal of treatment. Many neonatologists feel that the death of a baby in a neo-natal intensive care unit should not be seen as a failure, rather more as a baby who has died because of an untreatable condition but whose parents have been given the opportunity to know and love it.

Numbers

So how will the number of people with impairments and who are disabled by these, change over the years? In the United States, 2.6% of children under 3 years, 5.2% of children between 3 and 5 years, and 12.4% of young people between 6 and 21 years of age, have disabilities. Add to this the 48.9 million adults with disabilities, outside nursing homes and other institutions, and there is a sizeable proportion of the population who potentially need oral care, some of it special care. There is a preponderance of males over females in these figures and considerable racial variation in those affected[11,12].

Changing demographic trends show that the number of older and very old people in many societies will increase in the early part of the next century. For very elderly people, despite the association with increasing prevalence and incidence of chronic diseases and disability, the evidence is that there has been an improvement in the management of the latter. This has come about through the appropriate use of equipment and support in the home, which can be effective in reducing disability.

At the other end of the age scale, survival of small babies born as early as 23 weeks brings with it, in some cases, impairment. Levene[13] forecasts that a baby born at 24 weeks has a 25% chance of survival, at 26 weeks 50% and at 28weeks, 90%. Such young, small babies need to be ventilated and they are prone to brain haemorrhage as well as necrotising enterocolitis. For the survivors, there is a 5% chance of severe disability and a 10–15% risk of impairment.

We know however, that many people with impairments now survive much longer than was the case a decade or two ago. Of those people with spina bifida 70–80% reach their 20th birthday; the average life expectancy for people with cystic fibrosis is 26 years; there has been a 400 per cent increase in survival from leukaemia since 1960. In 1954, many people with Down syndrome did not survive to two years of age: in the 1990s, people with this condition live to 55 years and older[11]. Survival is not without other, acquired impairments: Alzeimer's disease, leukaemia, and an increased likelihood of Hepatits B. As more children with disabilities grow out of the scope of care of paediatric dentists, there is an urgent need for more general dentists with special skills and experience[14].

Health costs

Economists need a robust definition of disability for, for example, providing clinical care for people with impairments including the appropriate selection of treatments, predictions on prognosis and the planning of long-term care. Planners need the information for policy development and insurance companies or defence organisations to help in settling compensation claims.

Predicting health costs associated with disability are, on the whole, based on trends in the prevalence of chronic diseases and disability. However, potential patient pool changes will depend on a number of factors. Impairment is not a static process but a dynamic one, heterogeneous and changing. In general, more health care money is spent on the larger proportion of people who have less severe impairments than on the smaller group of individuals with severe disability. This is despite the fact that this latter group has a more than three-fold higher individual health expenditure[18]. There are opportunity costs too – what cost does society bear by preventing people from taking part in productive tasks through barriers raised by ignorance and discrimination?[19]

In the future, there may be an increase in the heterogeneity of impairment but a trend towards less severe forms of disability. Preventive practises may, for example, reduce the mortality associated with cancer, but with a resultant increase in morbidity. Likewise, prevention of impairments that are associated with disability, for example, cerebral palsy, may result in a reduction in morbidity. Screening for impairments and all that implies for costs is another contentious area.

Oral health and care

Oral care is provided to people with impairments in a variety of ways as indicated in other chapters (Chapters 12–14).

Characteristics of the interface between people with impairments and dental services:

- fewer dental visits/longer intervals between visits
- limited physical access to dental buildings
- unwillingness of clinicians to provide care
- financial difficulties
- history of extractions
- emergency hospital (2°) care rather than planned community (1°) care
- treatment with sedation/general anaesthesia[14]

Although not written about extensively in the literature, the provision of oral health care services to this group of people has not consistently been of the highest quality. Many patients have received little more than extractions and there has been a high prevalence of unmet need despite the overall decline in the prevalence of dental caries in the general population (*Table 2*). The exception to this is where dental services, often community-based, have been targeted on children with impairments (*Table 3*).

Table 2. Mean caries experience (DMFT) in children with physical disabilities (10–14-year-olds) in 1981 and 1990.

Caries experience (DMFT)	1981	1990
DMFT = 0	24%	51%
DMFT	1.9	2.1
D/DMFT %	37%	66%
M/DMFT %	26%	5%
F/DMFT %	37%	28%

Nunn and Murray 1987[15]; Nunn *et al* 1993[16]

Table 3. Comparison of mean DMFT values 1977–1982 in 13-year-old children in 'special schools'.

Caries experience (DMFT)	1977	1982
Number	106	49
DMFT	5.9	5.0
D	3.8	0.4
M	1.4	0.8
F	0.7	3.8
Service used:		
Community		80%
General/Private practice		20%
Hospital		–

Mellor and Doyle, 1987[17]

The poorer oral health of people with impairments is attributable to a number of causes[12]. In part, lack of awareness of the need for oral care, by parents or carers of a person with limited or no communication, contributed to emergency dental visits. This resulted in extraction of teeth and the slow transition to edentulousness in a patient who would not cope with the wearing of prostheses. Dentists for their part are not always able or willing to provide dental care for patients whom they regard as difficult. Too often patients are labelled as 'special needs' when all that this means is ordinary needs not ordinarily being met.

The reasons given by dentists for not providing services for people with impairments are:

- too time-consuming/expensive
- difficulties of access to the surgery
- challenging behaviour
- waiting room disturbances
- need for special facilities
- lack of training and experience[14,20]

Whilst there is little or no evidence to justify these claims, these issues are perceived by dentists as real and need to be addressed *(Figure 1)*[20].

For dentists working in a general practice, cost is perceived as a real barrier to providing services. In the UK, dentists working in their own practices in the National Health Service are paid a capitation fee for looking after children. This fee is doubled if the child has a disability. However, as *Table 4* shows, this has not resulted in an increased number of children with a disability who are looked after in general practice. Complementing this form of care is a salaried service that has a duty to provide care for all those people who are unable or unwilling to obtain their care through the general practice system. However, this service has suffered a significant reduction in staff such that, in 1985 there were 1.092 clinical dental officers, in 1990 there were 815 and by 1994 this had reduced to 649[21].

Alongside this, the 'Care in the Community' normalisation policy (see

Table 4. Number of children with disabilities registered with general dental practititioners (GDPs) in the UK 1991–1999

	March 1991	March 1996	March 1999
Number of children with disabilities registered	16,088	16,632	12,130
Total number of children registered	4,077,000	6,988,000	7,381,379

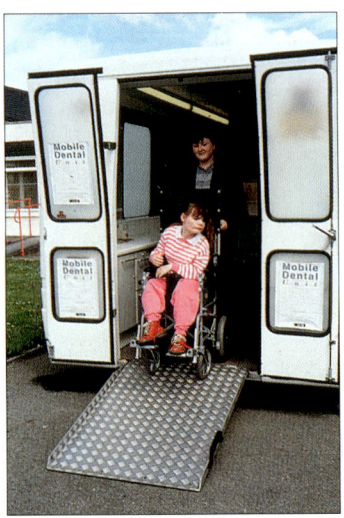

Figure 2

Mobile dental unit at an adult training centre to provide comprehensive care for clients

chapter 15) has meant that as clients have been rehoused out of long-stay residential hospitals and into care homes in local communities, they have lost contact with services traditionally provided by the hospital. The salaried community service has attempted to fulfil its role by offering care to people with disabilities in adult training centres. However, on occasions they have been turned away since the specialist service they wish to provide from mobile units (*Figure 2*) is seen as running contrary to the principle of 'normalisation'. Yet dentists in their local community have been unwilling to provide care for such people. On the limited evidence available, adults with intellectual impairments who have moved into independent living from long stay institutions have shown an increase in caries levels as their length of stay in the community increases. This is despite equity of access and an initially lower prevalence of caries compared with the general population[12].

When members of the dental team are asked what help they need in order to feel confident in providing care to people with impairments, education and training rank high.

Parents and carers

Garwick *et al.*[22] encapsulate what we need to bear in mind when caring for people with disabilities:

> *"You know this mother or father or whoever is with this person 24 hours a day knows more about this child than you ever will. You need to listen to what they are saying"*

Parents of children born with impairment have to go through a process akin to bereavement; these emotions cover grief – for the normal child they do not have, shock of coping with the unexpected, despair at the hopelessness of the situation, guilt, blame and anger for what they as parents may or may not have done. Or indeed, how the impairment may impact on future generations. These emotions may be followed by a state of detachment when life seems empty and meaningless. After a period of withdrawal, parents may come to accept their 'different' child and to make adjustments to a very different type of future to the one they had anticipated, accompanied by a sense of realism and even hope[23]. Whilst there is little evidence to support the view that the presence or type of disability increases the risk of family separation, it is a fact that maternal psychological health suffers; mothers tend to be the major care-givers and a father's employment outside the home may afford much need respite[24].

Here is one parent's view, who has an only child with cerebral palsy, now aged 16:

'In the early days following the birth of a child who has been brain damaged, parents do not function as normal parents might. The shock, grief and ongoing sense of bereavement for what has been lost added to the practical problems and major issues surrounding your child force dental health and hygiene low down on your scale of priorities. As so often is the case, it is only an issue when problems arise.'......... 'As well as the physical problems that toothache would present yet more pain for a child who has been through so much, how could he tell us where the pain was? The cosmetic issue of dental hygiene has always been important to us; when Alexander was young an educational psychologist told us that because he was a good-looking, responsive child, people would be attracted to him and this would be a great benefit. This has proved to be true. We have noticed the problem other, older children with cerebral palsy have with gaps, crooked, broken or discoloured teeth and the way people shun them or avoid contact.'

For siblings in the family it can be a time of emotional instability with a disproportionate amount of time devoted to the care of the child with impairments as well as a degree of isolation of the family within their local community. Adolescents with impairments are more likely to experience behavioural problems. How does the teenager with a 'hidden' impairment, a congenital heart defect for example, cope with the stress of daily living as compared to a child with cerebral palsy and in a wheelchair. Some disabilities, those involving the brain, for example epilepsy, engender more negative impact on the family. Families too have to cope with the stress of uncertainty: will the disease go into remission, for example, a child with cancer. How do they cope with unpredictable seizures? How do you come to terms with impairments where the prognosis is changing, as in cystic fibrosis?[11]

Children and adults with a disability are at greater risk of abuse; children with disabilities are twice as likely to be sexually abused and conversly, abused children are five times more likely to be intellectually impaired. Females are more vulnerable than males.

Factors associated with increased risk of abuse for a person with an impairment:

- dependent on others for needs
- lack of control or choice over own life
- compliance seen as desirable – equates with reward normally
- lack of knowledge about sex
- inability to differentiate different types of touching
- inability to communicate events
- mild versus severe impairment – reduces acceptance/less family support
- depersonalisation of the individual – less 'human', gives license to abuse[24]

For many parents the prospect that their disabled child will outlive them is real but there is reluctance on the part of parents to allow siblings to take over a care-giving role. Care of an elderly relative is usually a short-lived experience; in the US on average five years. By contrast caring for young, impaired offspring may occupy 50 or 60 years. The costs involved are significant. Again in the US, these can be as much as $6,400 per annum for a child with intellectual impairment.

For many older people with disabilities the prospect, after leaving formal education, is that they will live at home; in the US no more than 20% of people with intellectual impairment live in institutions. For many people with a disabled person living at home, services are worse; there is less respite care, financial help or counselling for family members.

These parents underline how self-reliant they have to be:

> 'As parents of Scott, a severely disabled 17-year-old (C.P.), life in general is an uphill struggle. A case of who shouts the loudest wins, a constant fight for one thing or another to get what's best for all of us. For most services to us, waiting months for appointments or equipment. As an example 'wheelchair services' can take up to a year to assess and deliver a wheelchair, another year to put right any adaptations, by which time Scott has grown and the procedure starts all over again.

> We have been in the position to help ourselves financially, buy the equipment ourselves, and therefore have less hassle.

> The dental service Scott receives is both caring and professional and supportive to us. It is the least trying and stressful than all the other services encountered.

> Scott is an only child and therefore we are able to commit totally to him in all areas and when appointments and meetings are made.

Finally we are very lucky to have a very close and supportive family, who are the best service to us!'

Dental educational needs

The foregoing underlines the need for members of oral health care teams to undertake further education and training in the effective dental care of people with impairments since it would appear that current undergraduate training is inadequate in this respect. When the FDI conducted its survey on the 'Oral health of the Handicapped' in 1989, less than half the member countries responding (n=54 countries) had any provision for under- or post-graduate training in the care of people with impairments. Nearly three quarters of those responding said that there were insufficient post-graduate seminars in the subject[25].

In a number of countries it is possible to obtain postgraduate training in the comprehensive delivery of care for people who have impairments. In the United States, Canada and Sweden for example, Hospital Dentistry is a recognised speciality and provides care for many compromised patients of all ages[26]. In the UK there are a number of University Masters programmes as well as a Royal College Diploma[27] providing training for specialists, the majority of whom will provide care in a primary, community-based setting. The latter UK-based programme, for which the first examination will take place in the year 2000, is expected to attract candidates from many parts of the world. Similarly there are courses as well as an examination designed especially for dental nurses in the same field of expertise.

Summary

However we choose to define disability in the years to come, people with impairments are increasingly raising their profile within society through advocacy and slowly changing attitudes on the part of communities, bullied to an extent by slow-moving legislation. Increasing numbers of people with impairments mean that their needs can no longer be denied particularly by so-called caring professions. The evidence that behaviour, well-being and appearance are improved by good oral care and thus social acceptability enhanced, is irrefutable. The dental team have a role and a duty to provide that care.

References

1. World Health Organization. *International Classification of impairments, disabilities and handicaps; a manual of classification relating to the consequences of disease.* World Health Organization, Geneva, 1980.

2. World Health Organization. *International Classification of impairments, Activities and Participation. A manual of dimensions of disablement and functioning. Beta 1 draft for field trials.* World Health

Organization, Geneva, 1997.

3. Vygotsky. *The collected works of Vygotsky. Vol 2: The Fundamentals of Defectology (Abnormal Psychology and Learning Disabilities)*. Ed: RW Rieber, AS Carlton. Plenum Press, New York. 1993.

4. Hutchison T. The classification of disability. *Arch Dis Child* 1995;**73**: 91–99.

5. Mehlman M J, Neuhauser D. Alternative definitions of disability: changes in a dichotomous v continuous system. *Dis Rehab* 1999;**21**: 385–387.

6. Kirchner C. Looking under the lamp post: inappropriate uses of measures just because they are there. *J Dis Policy Studies* 1996;**7**: 71–90

7. *Disability Discrimination Act. Code of Practice; Rights of Access to Goods, Facilities, Services and Premises.* Her Majesty's Stationery Office, London. 1999.

8. Waldman H B, Swerdloff M, Perlman SP. Children with mental retardation grow older. *J Dent Child* 1999; **66**: 266–272.

9. Devlieger P J. From handicap to disability: a language use and cultural meaning in the United States. *Dis Rehab* 1999; **7**: 346–354.

10. Barr O. Genetic counselling: a consideration of the potential and key obstacles to assisting parents adapt to a child with learning disabilities. *Br J Learn Dis* 1999; **27**: 30–36.

11. Waldman H B, Perlman S P, Swerdloff M. Children with disabilities: more than just numbers. *J Dent Child* 1999; **66**: 192–196.

12. Waldman H B, Perlman S P, Swerdloff M. Dental care for children with mental retardation: thoughts about the Americans with Disabilites Act. *J Dent Child* 1999; **65**: 487–491.

13. Levene M. In: *Too young to live, too small to die.* Ed: Cuffe J. The Times, 1992.

14. Waldman H B, Perlman S P, Swerdloff M. What if dentists did not treat people with disabilities? *J Dent Child* 1998; **65**: 96–101.

15. Nunn J H, Murray J J. The dental health of handicapped children in Newcastle and Northumberland. *Br Dent J* 1987; **162**: 9–14.

16. Nunn J H, Gordon P H, Carmichael C. Dental health status and unmet treatment need amongst children in special education. *Community Dent Health* 1993; **10**: 389–396.

17. Mellor J, Doyle A J. The evaluation of a dental treatment service for children attending special schools. *Community Dent Health* 1987; **4**: 43–48.

18. Kriegsman D M, Deeg D J H. Implications of alternative definitions of disability beyond health care expenditures. *Dis Rehab* 1999; **21**: 388–391.

19. Nunn J H, Murray J J. Dental care of handicapped children by general dental practitioners. *J Dent Educ* 1988; **52**: 463–465.

20. Oliver C H, Nunn J H. The accessibility of dental treatment to adults with physical disabilities aged 16–64 in the North-East of England. *Spec Care Dent* 1995; **15**:97–101.

21. Murray J J, Nunn J H. Trends in the Community Dental Service 1980–1990. *Community Dent Health* 1993; **10**:335–342.

22. Garwick A W, Kohrman C, Wolman C. Families' recommendations for improving services for children with chronic conditions. *Arch Paediatr Adolesc Med* 1998; **152**: 440–448.

23. Hirst M. Dissolution and reconstruction of families with a disabled young person. *Dev Med Child Neurology* 1991; **33**: 1073–1079.

24. Waldman H B, Perlman S P, Swerdloff M. A "dirty secret": the abuse of children with disabilities. *J Dent Child* 1999; **66**: 197–202.

25. Fédération Dentaire Internationale. Commission on Research and Epidemiology Report: Working Group 11. FDI, 1992.

26. Jolly D E, Martin M D, Brody H A, Glassman P D. Curriculum guidelines for the training of general practice residents in treating the patient with special needs. *Spec Care Dent* 1987; **7**: 150–153.

27. The Royal College of Surgeons of Edinburgh. *Regulations relating to the Diploma of Membership in Special Needs Dentistry (M SND.RCSEd).* Royal College of Surgeons of Edinburgh, Scotland, 2000.

Chapter 2

Barriers, Discrimination and Prejudice

Nick Watson

Introduction

It is estimated that there are around 500 million disabled people world wide, the largest number of whom is to be found in the Majority World. There is, however, a higher prevalence of disabled people in the wealthier nations. Advances in medical science and new medical interventions, which prolong life, coupled with demographic changes in the age of the population, suggest that these numbers will increase in the future. The implications of this in terms of social and economic policy will be far reaching. This chapter will briefly examine how organisations of disabled people have demanded, and to some extent achieved, a rethinking of what it means to be a disabled person. They have argued that disabled people should be seen as a minority group, as a group who face discrimination and oppression and that this discrimination and oppression is the result of the way that society is organised and not as a consequence of their impairment.

Numbers of people who are disabled will increase because of:

- enhanced survival
- more sophisticated medical care
- increased longevity

The meaning of disability and the personal consequences on individual lives of being a disabled person have changed considerably in the last twenty years. Prior to the 1970s the majority of disabled people, in most of the Western world at least, would have been found in large isolated, residential establishments. Employment opportunities for many were restricted to special 'training centres' or sheltered employment with an emphasis on work as rehabilitation. These centres typically offered poor training, little opportunity for advancement and low wage levels. Disabled children were segregated from their non-disabled peers and, under the guise of rehabilitation, denied access to a full curriculum, spending much of their time in physiotherapy. This in turn served to deny them future opportunities. Disabled people were also denied sexual rights, the rights to form relationships, reproductive rights and the right to lead independent lives. Whilst these conditions still exist for many disabled people, increasing numbers have been able to access mainstream employment, mainstream schooling, live independently in the community, form relationships and have children. The fact that some can do it suggests that all should be able to do it and that they are held back by social, economic and political factors rather than their impairment.

Features of the lives of people with disability in the 1970s and 1980s:

- residential care
- Special schools
- adult training centres
- day centres

Challenging the understanding of disablement

The traditional way to view disablement is to see it simply as a medical problem. Disability, in this approach, and the problems faced by disabled people arise as a result of their impairment. For example people would say, "She is disabled because she has epilepsy", or "He is disabled because he broke his back"[1]. This is what is called the medical or individual model and is the basis for both current medical treatment of disabled people and the many approaches to disability that utilise the World Health Organization's International Classification of Impairments, Disabilities and Handicaps. Put simply this schema suggests that impairments are the result of a biological or psychological abnormality, that disabilities are the resulting restrictions in activity and that handicaps are the disadvantages faced by disabled people that arise as a result of impairments or disabilities. Impairment is therefore seen as the cause of the disadvantages faced by disabled people.

Medical model:

- Impairment – abnormality, defect, condition
- Disability – restriction of activity as a consequence of impairment
- Handicap – disadvantage suffered because of impairment and disability

It is an individualistic approach, one which presents impairment as the 'all'[2]. The individual disabled person becomes the centre of attention and the focus is on changing the individual, usually through the modification of their impairment. The focus is on cure and rehabilitative medical intervention. Through this reification of impairment, control over the lives of disabled people moves to the medical profession. If disablement can only be cured through medical intervention, it follows that the fortunes of disabled people lie in the hands of the medical profession (regardless of whether or not the medical profession can treat a particular impairment). The medical 'expert' defines what it is that an individual needs, how these needs should be met and how the negative consequences of an individual's disability can be minimised[3].

Autonomy is removed and the picture of a disabled person as one who is a victim of their impairment emerges, what Oliver[2] has called 'the personal tragedy theory of disability'.

In addition, as Barnes and his colleagues[3] point out, the medical model, by linking impairment with disability presents the environment as 'neutral' and stable. The possibility of changing environments and thus removing barriers is ignored. These authors also suggest that in the medical model the onus be on the individual to adapt, to adopt coping strategies and to limit their own hopes and ambitions.

In the late 1960s and 1970s disabled people throughout the world began to organise, to challenge their isolation and to demand equal rights. In doing so they also challenged the individual medical model of disability. Organisations such as the Union of the Physically Impaired Against Segregation (UPIAS) in the United Kingdom, the Independent Living Movement in America and the Handicappenförbundens Centralkommitté in Sweden all called for an alternative approach to disability. The UPIAS document, The Fundamental Principles of Disability, published in 1976[4], laid the foundations for what Oliver[2] later called the social model of disability. Put simply this approach argues that it is society which disables people with impairment by its failure to include them. Society, it is argued, is responsible for the creation of disability through social, cultural and environmental barriers; 'In our view it is society which disables physically impaired people. Disability is something which is imposed on top of our impairments by the way we are unnecessarily isolated and excluded from full participation in society. Disabled people are therefore an oppressed group in society'[4]. The rejection of any link between impairment and disability has been adopted by the majority of organisations of disabled people throughout the world. Disabled People International have adopted the following definition:

Social Model:
- IMPAIRMENT: is the functional limitation within the individual caused by physical, mental or sensory impairment.
- DISABILITY: is the loss or limitation of opportunities to take part in the normal life of the community on an equal level with others due to physical and social barriers.

In this approach, not being able to walk would be seen as an impairment, whilst being denied access to a building through the presence of steps is a disability. The social model moves the attention from an individual's impairment to the external environment in which they are situated and the obstacles imposed on disabled people. It is society which disables people with impairments and the way to ameliorate disability is to change society, not the individual. Disablement has nothing to do with an individual's impairment, but is the result of

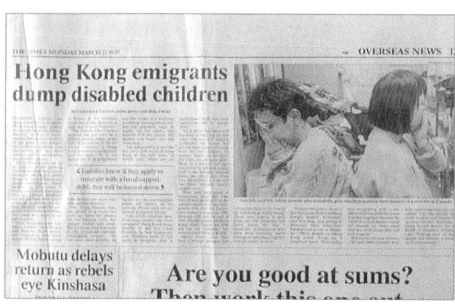

social oppression[5]. Implicit in this approach to disability is the idea that disabled people are the best experts on their own lives.

This political shift in the definition of disability has led to an upsurge in the consciousness of disabled people, the formation of new self-organised groups, and campaigns for anti-discrimination legislation and independent living. New techniques, such as direct action, and new forms of cultural expression, such as disability arts, have accompanied new ways of identifying and organising.

What are the barriers?

The barriers that disabled people face can be divided into two broad categories: those arising from discrimination and those arising from prejudice (*Figure 1*). Discriminatory barriers include those that physically exclude disabled people such as stairs rather than lifts, the absence of disabled toilets, heavy doors, poor lighting or high counters. These barriers also include those of a more structural nature. For example Barnes *et al.*[3] document how educational attainment for the many disabled children that are educated in segregated schools is below that of their non-disabled peers and they experience a narrower curriculum. Consequently they leave school with fewer academic skills and qualifications than their peers which limits their opportunities in later life.

Employment, as the same authors show, is another area where disabled people face exclusion. In the UK the unemployment rate for disabled people in 1995 was nearly three times that of non-disabled people. Similarly, a recent poll in the USA revealed that only 29 per cent of disabled adults are employed, as against a figure of 79 per cent among the non-disabled population. Furthermore, the majority of jobs open to disabled people tend to be low paid, low skilled jobs. Disabled men earn about a quarter less than there nondisabled counterparts.

Structural discrimination also exists in housing, in the provision of public transport, and in welfare and other social services. Barnes *et al.*[3] argue

Figure 2

A newspaper headline after a man was refused entry to Australia in order to join his family, on his retirement from the UK. The Australian Government felt that his diabetes could, potentially, impose a burden on the country's health resources long-term.

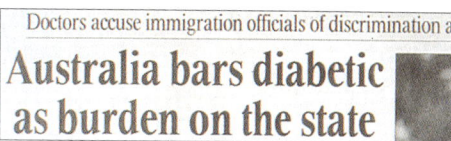

Doctors accuse immigration officials of discrimination a

Australia bars diabetic as burden on the state

that the systemic nature of the inequalities faced by disabled people has not been addressed by social policy initiatives. Such initiatives, they suggest have tended to focus on the individual as the problem rather than address the social and economic causes of the problem. At best these policy initiatives will simply fail to solve the problem they seek to address, at worse they will add to the problems faced by disabled people, as, for example in the case of special education.

Prejudice also presents barriers to the full participation in society by disabled people. Disabled people are subjected to stares, are placed at the centre of unwanted attention, are denied anonymity as they go about their day to day lives and are patronised. As Morris[6] in her aptly named book, *Pride Against Prejudice*, writes:

> *"It is not only physical limitations that restrict us to our homes and those whom we know. It is the knowledge that each entry into the public world will be dominated by stares, by condescension, by pity and by hostility."*
> *(p 25)*

Disabled people have an identity imposed upon them. It doesn't matter what they do, what their job is or what they say, what is important in the eyes of many is the fact that they are disabled. As a consequence non-disabled people feel free to stare at them, to make comments about their physical condition and deny them the respect they would accord to others.

When such an identity is fostered on to disabled people not only can this, as Morris[6] argues, impact on the way that people think about themselves, it also constrains opportunities for disabled people (*Figure 2*). For example Davis *et al.*[7] illustrate how the closed minds of some people working with severely disabled children limit not only their expectations of the child, but also what the child is willing to do. They show how, through employing what they term reflexivity when working with the children, that is self-analysis and political awareness, the children show much more ability and are more willing to co-operate and communicate. They argue that the key to meeting the challenge to working with these children is to examine your own

19

feelings and prejudices and how these impact on practice. The problems they suggest lie not with the child, but with the way that the child is treated.

Barriers:

- Discrimination
  – physical access to premises
  – lowered educational expectations
  – excluded from employment
  – social policies imposed
- Prejudice
  – unwanted centre of attention
  – denied anonymity
  – patronised
  – imposed identity
  – denied respect

Conclusion – implications for dentistry

As well as ensuring the physical accessibility of their premises, the dental team should start by examining their own practices and procedures, rather than assuming that it is only and always the disabled person who is the problem. For example, when dealing with people with a learning difficulty who exhibits what is termed challenging behaviour the question should be asked "Whose challenging behaviour, the dentists or the patient?"

Professionals should treat disabled people as agents who are capable of expressing views and having preferences, and they should try and meet these preferences wherever possible. This can raise some difficult issues. For example, do people with learning difficulties who do not want to go to the dentist have a right to opt to let their teeth decay? Or does the dentist and those who care for that person have a duty to ensure that the person has good teeth for their own good, regardless of that individual's wishes? These and other similar issues need to be addressed when providing care for disabled people and if they are to be successful then it is essential that the problem is located in the right place. Impairment is not the problem, it is the way that people with impairment are treated that is the problem.

References

1. Oliver M. *Understanding Disability: From theory to practice.* Macmillan, Basingstoke, 1996.
2. Oliver M. *The Politics of Disablement.* Macmillan, Basingstoke, 1990.
3. Barnes C, Mercer G and Shakespeare T. *Exploring Disability: A sociological introduction.* Polity Press, Cambridge, 1999.
4. UPIAS. *The fundamental principles of Disability.* London, Union of the Physically Impaired Against Segregation, 1976.
5. Thomas C. *Female Forms: Experiencing and understanding disability.* Open University Press, Buckingham, 1999
6. Morris J. *Pride Against Prejudice.* Women's Press, London, 1991
7. Davis J M, Watson N and Cunningham-Burley S. Learning the Lives of Disabled Children: Developing a reflexive approach. In Christensen P and James A (eds): *Conducting Research With Children.* Falmer, London, 2000.

Chapter 3

Consent: Making Decisions and Vulnerability

Jenny King

Introduction

Making clinical decisions with and for vulnerable others is never easy. There are complex ethical dilemmas in balancing the need to provide the necessary care whilst at the same time respecting autonomy, even if this may be limited. The related law has been described as, *'fragmented and unsatisfactory,'* and has been subject to change[1]. In clinical practice there are difficult judgements for the clinician to make and communication challenges. In any discussion of providing care for people who are vulnerable it is important to recognise these difficulties from the outset. Nevertheless moral reasoning and legal theory have deliberated these issues and provide some guidelines for clinicians treating vulnerable patients.

Much of what has been written about clinical decision making for vulnerable patients has considered general medical care, for example Brock and Buchanan's book *Deciding for Others*[2]. In dentistry the same principles apply[3]. However dentistry has some distinctive aspects. For example dental treatment is most often elective, and although emergencies, such as severe toothache, may occur, these are rarely life threatening. Furthermore dentists often build up long term relationships with patients and provide regular preventive and maintenance care over many years. Most dental treatment for people with impairments is simple routine dentistry, just like any other patient. However preventive care may be difficult for people who must rely on others for basic food choices and daily oral hygiene. Examples of those occasions where dentistry may present more complex decisions would be in the management of cleft palates and facial deformities.

Ways in which dentistry differs from medicine, as far as obtaining consent for intellectually impaired patients is concerned:

- Procedures are usually elective
- Dental 'emergencies' are rarely life-threatening
- Dentist:patient relationship is built up over years
- Most dental care is simple, routine and regular
- Patient may be reliant on others for maintenance and prevention

This chapter provides a brief overview of the ethical and legal considerations that inevitably arise for dentists when a vulnerable person needs dental treatment. Particularly it considers what is good practice in how treatment decisions are made, who has ultimate responsibility and the appropriate sharing of responsibilities.

The ethical principle of informed consent

Any understanding of decision making for people with physical or mental impairments should be thought about in the light of good consenting practice generally, whether this is a blind person attending the dental surgery with a cavity in a tooth, or an elderly edentulous woman on a geriatric ward. The widely accepted ethical principle of informed consent says that people should be informed, understand and not be coerced into treatment. Information should be given about the nature of the problem, the reason for any proposed treatment and any options including the option of no treatment. Any significant risks of treatment and the expected benefits should be discussed together with how long treatment might take and, if applicable, any costs.

Only if a person has a reasonable understanding of these aspects of treatment are they in a position to weigh up any advantages and disadvantages, make choices for themselves and give their consent to any particular treatment that the dentist proposes. Although these principles are not always put into practice in dentistry, and dentists frequently make paternalistic decisions on behalf of patients, informed consent and respect for patients rights is nevertheless the general moral context in which decisions about dental treatment for vulnerable patients must be considered[4,5].

Ethical principles of informed consent:
- be competent
- be informed
- understand
- not be coerced

Assessing competence

For many adults with physical impairments these will be the normal considerations for obtaining their consent to treatment, although there may sometimes be additional communication challenges. For example a person may have impaired hearing or a dentist and patient do not share the same culture or language. Many people with impairments are quite capable of making up their own minds about their dental treatment and giving their consent to treatment. Adults should always be assumed competent to give their own consent to dental treatment unless there is good reason to think otherwise.

However vulnerable adults may not always have the necessary capacity to consent to treatment for themselves. The first task for the dentist is therefore to decide at the outset if the person they are treating has the necessary ability to understand, reason, recall and apply to themselves the information and explanations given to them about their dental treatment. In legal terminology a dentist must judge whether or not the patient is competent to give their consent to treatment.

A learning difficulty does not of itself imply that a person is not legally competent. For instance a person with mild Down syndrome may well be judged to be competent to give their consent. In practice it may be quite clear to everyone concerned from ordinary conversational ability that a person cannot make their own decisions. In other situations it may not be so clear cut. This may be a difficult clinical judgement – although it may often not be the dentist who has to make these judgements. There is the danger either that a person is judged to be incompetent who would be able to consent for themselves, or a person may be judged to be competent when they are not[6].

Sometimes other clinicians may have already made a judgement about a persons competence or lack of it. For example a person who is in long term hospital care. But it is important to note that competence is task specific - that although a person may not be judged to be competent in one area of their lives (e.g. deciding about major surgery) this does not necessarily mean that they are not competent in another area (e.g. deciding about routine dental treatment).

A person's capacity to consent may be permanently or temporarily impaired. A patient born with severe Down syndrome may never be capable of consenting to treatment, whereas a person who is temporally irrational for psychiatric reasons may return to their normal competency. Decisions about elective dental care can be postponed until a patient recovers from temporary incompetence. In this context it should be noted that compulsory detainment for treatment of psychiatric illness does not mean that consent need not be obtained for any other medical or dental treatment if the patient is judged to be competent.

Attempts have been made to describe routines or 'competency tests' for assessing a person's capacity to give their consent, but for the reasons that have been outlined these are difficult to apply generally. For the most part a judgement about competency to consent must be made by the dentist providing treatment in the light of individual cases and situations.

Competence is:
- task specific
- variable from one occasion to another
- the responsibility of the clinician to decide

Who consents

If a patient is unable to consent for themselves then there is a question about the best treatment and who can decide and give the go ahead for treatment to proceed. What would be best for instance for a patient with learning difficulties who has lost a front tooth as a result of trauma suffered during an epileptic fit. Should the tooth be replaced with a denture, with a bridge or the gap left as it is?

With a child the situation is reasonably clear. Whether the child has an impairment or not the legal responsibility for consent rests with the parents. The usual principles of consent for children apply until a child reaches the age of medical consent. In most countries this is now set at the age of 16 or 18.

However the main focus of this discussion is on adults. The legal situation may vary in different countries. There are three possibilities for who takes responsibility for treatment to proceed: first relatives or carers acting as guardians, second responsible clinicians acting in the interests of patients, and third, as a last resort, the courts. None of these is without difficulty. But whoever makes the final decision the guiding principle must be that which is in the patients best interest, taking all the relevant considerations into account.

Relatives or carers

A vulnerable adult may continue to be dependent on their parents or other relatives for care and support beyond the age of maturity. Those who care for them on a day to day basis will know them very well and have a good idea of their capabilities and responses. Often such care is given at very considerable personal expense. Parents may for example give up paid employment in order to care for their vulnerable adult children unable to look after themselves. They are used to making decisions on behalf of the people that they look after. Respecting and taking into account the views of relatives when decisions must be made about dental care is important for the carer and the dentist too, since the patient will often be reliant on their family to support them both in preventive care at home and to bring them for dental appointments[7].

In other instances a person may be in long term residential care. Here decisions may be doubly difficult because both relatives and those carers responsible for everyday care will have an interest in any proposed treatment.

Whoever has the final responsibility in law for making any decisions, good practice must be to communicate with parents and carers as well as possible before any serious or irreversible decisions are made, for example giving a general anaesthetic or extracting a tooth. Most often the best interests of the patient are served by appropriate consultation. Although in cases where a person is in severe pain the patients best interests may be to go ahead with the extraction. But for all aspects of dental care the support of family and carers remains very important. Families and carers want to, and should be, involved in decision-making for those who depend on them for everyday care.

Clinicians

Clinicians are in a good position to make treatment decisions since they are the people most likely to be aware of the various options that are available and of any advantages or disadvantages of each option. Often clinicians who treat vulnerable patients specialise in their care and will have a broad perspective on what is possible and practical in managing different clinical situations. Their clinical knowledge and expertise gives them an overview which individual families may not have. Furthermore they are more likely to be neutral, although it can never be assumed that clinicians own interests will not enter the decision making process.

English law at present allows only clinicians to make decisions on behalf of incompetent adult patients. This means that no adult may consent for another adult, in other words there is no adult proxy for the purposes of dental care[8]. However this does not mean that clinicians should not consult with relatives, carers and patients themselves. It is also wise to consult with clinical colleagues when a decision is particularly serious or complex. However this does mean that asking a parent of an incompetent adult to sign a consent form for a general anaesthetic is not legally necessary, although it might well be good practice to seek the assent of relatives. Whatever the situation it is important for the responsible dentist to document how and why decisions were made about treatment for vulnerable patients.

The courts

In the English courts in a series of cases in the 1980s an attempt was made to establish who had responsibility for clinical decisions about sterilisation for sexually active women with learning disability. The judgement in a landmark case (F v West Berkshire 1989) that the decisions should rest with the responsible clinician has to some extent clarified the legal situation, although many writers and clinicians still consider this to be a grey and difficult area[8]. However, in the last resort, serious situations should be referred to the courts, particularly where there remains any dispute. In general good practice skills should prevent such cases ever reaching the courts.

Internationally the law may differ. There may for instance be various models of guardianship or substituted judgement in Europe and North America[9]. However national and international law regarding treatment for those with impaired decision making capacity is now under review. These legal differences reflect the very real difficulties of balancing the rights of patients and carers and the duties of clinicians in making decisions on behalf of others.

Good dental care should be available to vulnerable people in the same way as it is to any other patient. Decision making should be patient centred and not for the convenience of carers or clinicians[10]. But there is always a dilemma for clinicians providing dental care for vulnerable patients. On the one hand they do not want to neglect to provide the necessary treatment, whilst on the other hand they do not want to force treatment on an unwilling patient, even though that patient may have limited autonomy. An acceptable way must be found between neglect and abuse.

There can never be a perfect resolution to this dilemma, but a number of factors may help. In dentistry there is nearly always an option of waiting. A vulnerable adult who on one occasion may refuse to sit in the dental chair and have her mouth examined may on another day be quite prepared to co-operate. With patience, good communication and patient management skills many vulnerable people can be treated in the conventional way just as other patients are. Then there are times when carrying out the necessary treatment under general anaesthetic is the most appropriate course of action. The difficulty for the dentist is in deciding with others which will be the best management strategy for any particular person. However in the end the most important thing may be to make a decision and act on it. Many people with impairments have had their oral health seriously neglected because dentists have been afraid to proceed because of the perceived difficulties involved.

Patients with impairments may become subconsciously aware of any negative attitudes, even though they may not be directly expressed, and this is likely to affect their willingness to co-operate. Good practice entails positive attitudes, building up good relationships from the start, not rushing into treatment before patients and carers have become familiar with the clinical environment, instituting good preventive care so that intervention is minimised, ensuring long term continuity of regular maintenance care, making sure that time is taken for good communication, and giving attention to the necessary consultation and sharing of responsibilities. These will all contribute to reducing the number of times that serious conflicts about consent arise.

'Good Practice' entails:

- Allowing the opportunity for optimal co-operation – return another day if necessary
- Patience
- Good communications
- good patient management skills
- Making appropriate decisions
- Preventing disease to minimise interventions
- Providing regular maintenance care
- Forming a partnership with patient, family and carers

Those dentists who spend time treating vulnerable patients know both how difficult it can be but also what, with care, can be achieved, and how rewarding that is.

Consider the following case:-

A fifty year old woman who lives in a residential home develops a tooth ache. She has no relatives other than her elderly mother who visits her once a month. A care worker contacts your clinic and asks you to see her. The following day she attends the clinic with her care worker. The care worker tells you that she needs help with washing and dressing and that she cannot go out alone as she wanders off and gets lost. She has lived in the home for the past 20 years. She tells you her name is Mary de Souza but she is easily distracted and her conversation is limited and disjointed. However she is quite co-operative and allows you to examine her mouth. She has been to the dentist on several previous occasions. The tooth causing her pain has a large cavity. In your view it could be either filled or extracted.

The first decision you must make is whether or not she is legally competent to consent to treatment herself. She clearly cannot live an independent life and her conversation suggests that her ability to reason and understand is very limited. Her learning difficulty is quite severe and you record in your clinical records that she is not competent to decide for herself about how this tooth should be treated. (note that competence is task specific, she may be able to consent to other things. For example she may agree to sit in the dental chair and have her mouth examined)

Having decided that she is not legally competent to give her own consent it then remains to decide who should give legal consent. In some countries a relative or guardian may consent, in others proceeding with treatment is the responsibility of the clinician who acts in the patients best interests. But whatever the national law good ethical practice is for clinicians to inform and consult with appropriate others. In this case this might include care workers in the residential home, her elderly mother, and a second clinical opinion may be sought from another dentist or doctor. The patient herself should be given a simple explanation and her views sought as far as she is able to express them. Pain relief should be the first consideration and control of any infection. It is often better not to rush into any irreversible treatment, but to take time to discuss the best way forward. Once treatment for the toothache is completed then arrangements should be made for her continuing regular dental care.

Summary and conclusions

Vulnerable people deserve the best possible care, but it must be acknowledged that providing dental care for vulnerable patients is never easy. The difficulties that arise often relate to decision making, communication, co-operation and consent, rather than to any of the clinical technicalities of dental treatment. Dentists must make judgements about a patient's competency and also about what treatment is right for the patient. Having a good understanding of the ethical and legal issues that are raised and always applying good consenting practice will help the dentist to feel more confident when facing the dilemmas of a particular situation. Although the details of the law may be specific to any one country, the ethical considerations that have been discussed remain the same. The possibility of more shared responsibility in decision making, in consultation with relatives, carers and colleagues, whilst involving patients to the extent that they are able, offers a positive way forward. Continuity of care and respect for the rights, dignity and autonomy of patients and their carers, form the basis for good professional practice which will be both ethically and legally acceptable in providing dental care for those who are vulnerable.

References

1. Luttrell S. Making Decisions about medical treatment for mentally incapable adults in the UK. *Lancet* 1997; **350**: 950–953.
2. Buchanan A, Brock D. *Deciding for Others*. Cambridge University Press, 1989.
3. Shuman S, Berbeau M. Ethical and Legal Issues in Special Patient Care. *Dent Clin N Am* 1994; **38**: 553–557.
4. Ferguson F, Cinotti D, Kin W, Berensten B. Facilitation of informed consent for agency residents with developmental disabilities. *Spec Care Dent* 1996; **16**: 15–17.
5. Odom J, Odom S, Jolly D. Informed consent and the geriatric dental patient. *Spec Care Dent* 1992;
    12: 202–206.
6. Backler P. Assessing decision making capacity is a slippery business. *Community Ment Health J* 1996; **32**: 321–325.
7. Brock D. What is the moral authority of family members to act as surrogates for incompetent patients? *Milbank Quarterly* 1996; **74**: 599–618.
8. Brazier M. *Medicine Patients and the Law*. Penguin, 1993; pp 94–101.
9. Blankman K. Guardianship models in the Netherlands and Western Europe. *Int J Law Psychiatry* 1997; **20**: 47–57.
10. Brock D. Good decision making for incompetent patients. *Hastings Centre Report* 1994; **24**: S8–11.

Chapter 4

Practical Prevention

Bitte Ahlborg

Introduction

It is important for the physical and mental condition of a seriously ill or disabled patient to have a clean and healthy mouth. Therefore, oral care is a part of the daily routine in nursing, though often difficult to carry out especially if the patient cannot co-operate.

The oral cavity is a most private part of the body. This can be the reason why some anxious and confused patients do not want to be helped with their oral care. Another reason can be fear of pain. Therefore, it is of great importance to treat the patient in a kind and considerate way with respect for their integrity.

Need for good oral care for ill and disabled patients

Patients in poor health have little resistance to infections and easily sustain damage to the oral mucous membranes. Good oral hygiene is of the utmost importance in curing or relieving symptoms in the mouth.

Reasons for difficulties in managing oral hygiene without help or support:

- bad general condition because of a serious illness
- mental depression for a long time
- poor motor control of the cheeks, lips and tongue caused by paralysis or weakness
- dysfunction in arms and hands
- dry mouth with thick ropy mucus or crusts which complicate cleaning

Many persons with serious or chronic diseases have considerably reduced salivary secretion. An important property of saliva is to lubricate and protect the oral mucous membrane. A dry mucous membrane is fragile and can easily be damaged. Sores and fissures will be infected by bacteria or fungus. Conditions like these can be very painful and make it difficult to eat. In addition, reduced salivation implies a high risk of dental caries.

Furthermore thirst, as well as 'eating for consolation' or 'comfort eating', result in caries and dental erosion because of frequent intake of acid sweets and drinks.

Accordingly, there are several reasons for bad oral health because of disabilities or diseases. These call for special care in preventive dentistry.

Preventive measures for patients who run a high risk of caries and periodontal diseases

The three cornerstones in preventive dentistry for high-risk patients of all ages are fluorides, good oral hygiene and a well thought-out diet. It is often very difficult to alter the habits of diet and eating as well as to improve the oral hygiene, but it is never impossible to add fluorides of any kind.

Fluorides

Small quantities of fluoride applied frequently and on a regular basis can strengthen the enamel and prevent caries in high risk patients. Fluorides will also have an effect on exposed root surfaces of the teeth and therefore be of great importance in elderly people who run the risk of developing root caries.

The most common way to administer fluorides is through toothpaste, but there are several other forms of individual fluoride application. Fluoride varnish is a particularly useful form of topical fluoride since its application does not require prolonged isolation of the dental arches and it is tolerant of moisture, setting under saliva. Dental hygienists may carry out professional preventive fluoride programs in the dental clinics.

If administration of fluorides in tablets is used in children, the level of fluoride in drinking water must be taken into account when deciding dosage. Many disabled young people will not be able to comply with the normal regime of fluoride tablet use, that is, allowing the tablet to dissolve slowly in their mouth so that fluoride drops may be more acceptable.

For the disabled person who cannot tolerate toothpaste intra-orally then carers may consider using a toothbrush dipped in fluoride mouthwash (0.05% sodium fluoride [250ppm F⁻] or 0.2% sodium fluoride [1000ppm F⁻] in order to ensure daily contact of fluorides with the teeth.

Oral hygiene

When a patient with lowered resistance has advanced periodontal disease this must be treated promptly. Every time the patient bites or chew, a bacteraemia will be induced and this can affect the persons overall health. There is good evidence in the literature now to link periodontal disease and heart conditions. Hard and soft aggregations of bacteria on tooth surfaces and mucous membranes of the mouth will increase the risk of periodontal disease, candidosis, dental caries and a general feeling of discomfort.

Dental staff must clean the mouth by removing calculus and dental plaque, excavating caries and restoring the teeth either with temporary or permanent fillings. Sometimes the treatment calls for co-operation with the patients physician, in some cases antibiotics will be necessary before carrying out extractions, scaling or any other surgical procedures.

Diet

The risk of caries increases if the patient has to eat or drink frequently, especially if the food or fluid contains sugar. Many disabled patients have feeding difficulties and fail to gain weight . These patients may be taking high calorie, possible high sugar-containing, supplements which may be very cariogenic. A balance must be struck between maintaining good oral health and ensuring that the patient thrives. Some child patients may fail to thrive and may be fed by nasogastric tube but more usually by a gastrostomy, so that food enters the stomach directly, by-passing the mouth. Such children tend not to develop dental caries but rather to accumulate significant quantities of calculus.

If the patient's condition or state of health permits the most appropriate advice will be:

- Regular mealtimes – 4–5 meals a day
- Fresh water or mineral water to drink between meals
- Food that encourages chewing in order to increase saliva stimulation

Dental care for patients with natural teeth

In order to carry out a proper cleaning, it is important to be able to make a good inspection of the oral cavity. The patient sometimes needs support to get relaxation of the muscles of the face and jaws and a relaxed body posture.

The caregiver should either stand up or sit down beside/behind the patient (*Figure 1*).

A soft toothbrush with a small head is recommended as well as a systematic tooth-brushing technique (*Figures 2–4*).

There are a number of various aids available for interdental cleaning (*Figure 5*).

Daily fluoride application is one of the most efficient preventive

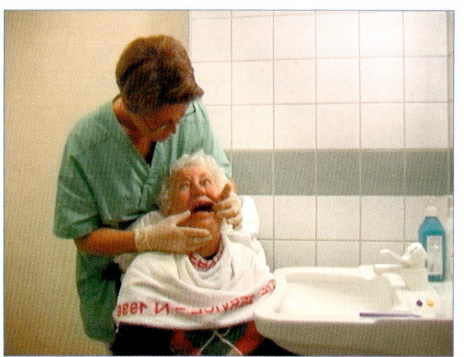

Figure 1

Standing beside the patient, the caregiver places her left arm around the back of the patient's head as a support and uses her left hand to keep the mouth open in order to get a sufficient view of the oral cavity

Figure 2

Bring down the lower lip with left thumb and hold the hand around the chin. Brush the front teeth of the lower jaw.

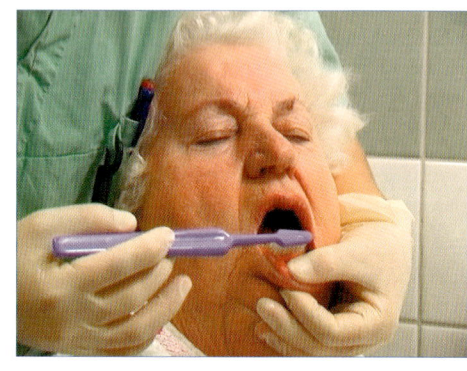

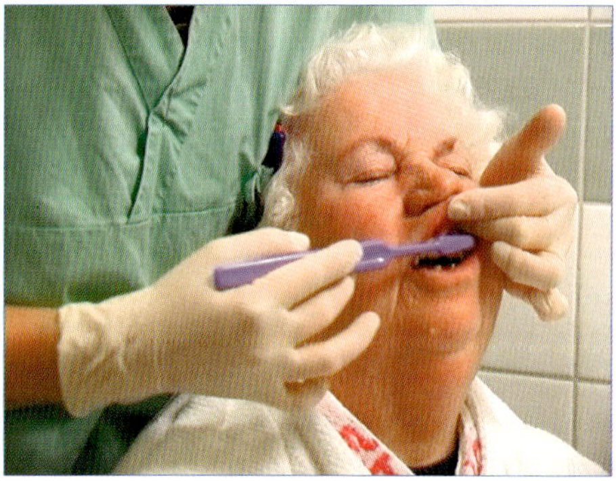

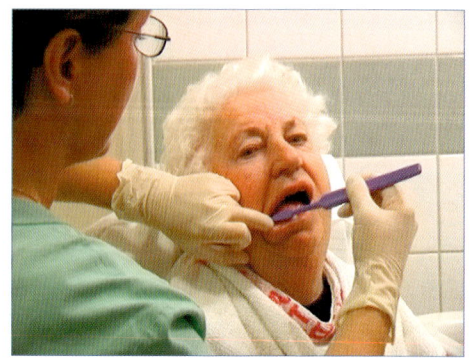

Figure 3

Bring up the upper lip with left forefinger and brush the front teeth of the upper jaw.

Figure 4

Stand up or sit down in front of the patient. Hold out right cheek with left forefinger and brush the teeth of the right upper- and lower jaw.

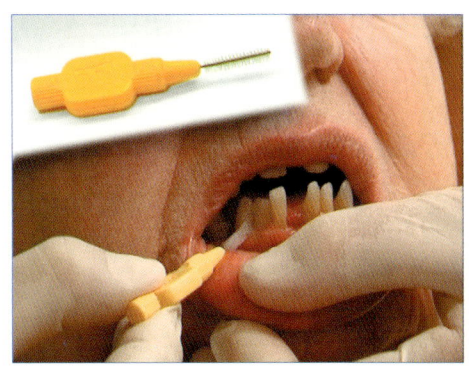

Figure 5

These special inter-dental brushes are very easy to handle and a good example of an effective technical aid for this purpose.

measures against dental caries and should be used in the mouth care programme.

Chlorhexidine can sometimes be prescribed by the dentist or the dental hygienist in order to complete, or to compensate for the brushing of teeth, for example, the need for high quality oral hygiene when the patient for some reason cannot carry out mechanical cleaning.

When chlorhexidine is prescribed and the patient is incapable of rinsing, swabbing with the solution is a good way of application. There are also other methods of administration, for example chlorhexidine gel 1% used as toothpaste or in individually made soft plastic trays. Alternatively, the hygienist or dentist may apply chlorhexidene varnish to the gingival margins for a sustained effect within the gingival crevice.

Chlorhexidine is the drug of choice in selected cases. This treatment should start with an examination of the oral cavity in order to do some primary cleaning, e.g. scaling and polishing teeth, cleaning mucous membranes and tongue.

It is essential to test the daily mouth-care yourself. Therefore technical aids must be tested and adjusted to the ability of the patient.

Oral care of seriously ill or unconscious patients

The aims of mouth care for the very ill can be classified as:
- Maintenance of comfort
- Cleanliness
- Moistening
- Prevention of infection

The following is a regime for carrying out daily oral care:
- Prepare by placing the necessary equipment on the table beside the patient.

33

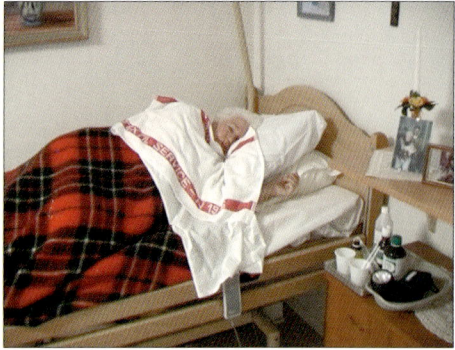

Figure 6

The patient in a proper position in order to avoid aspiration.

Figure 7

This bite-support of plastic is held by the index- or long-finger and put between the jaws in order to help the patient to keep the mouth open.

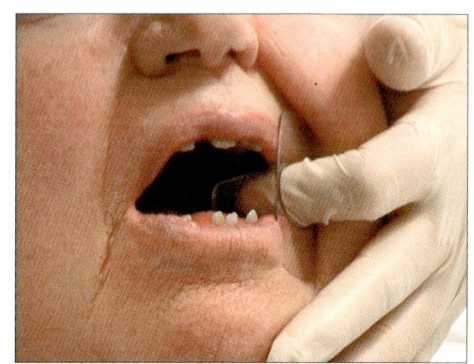

- Turn the patient on to their side.
- Place a towel or cellulose wadding under the chin (*Figure 6*).
- If the patient is unconscious the dentures should be removed whenever there is any risk that they will loosen and obstruct the oropharynx.

It is strongly recommended that two personnel carry out the oral care if the patient is unconscious. One of them assists while the other one carefully cleans the mouth and teeth. If there is a risk that the patient may suddenly bite together, the mouth can be held open by use of a bite-support (*Figure 7*).

The mucous membranes are moistened with water-dipped swabs (*Figure 8*).

Any existing mucus or crust on the tongue, in the palate or at the teeth can be dissolved with mucolytic solvent, for example ***Bisolvon® 2 mg/ ml (drips) (bromhexin hydrocloride)***. Dip a swab or a soft toothbrush alternately in this solvent and water (*Figure 9*).

When the patient has natural teeth, these should be cleaned in a mechanical and/or chemical way.

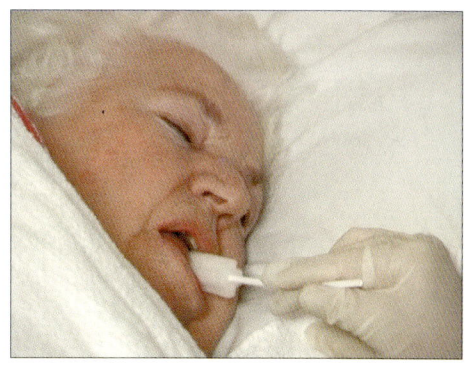

Figure 8

A foam stick applicator is a very useful aid for oral care

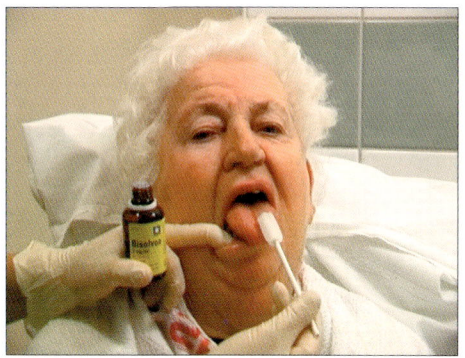

Figure 9

A tongue with a covering of dry debris and bacterial aggregation is to be cleaned. It is important to be careful and try to avoid initiating the vomiting-reflex

If the patient suffers from dry mouth it is important to wet the oral cavity with water as often as possible or at least every second hour. Alternatively a salivary substitute or lubricating solutions can be used. Care must be taken to select the most appropriate saliva substitute in order to avoid those which contain citric acid that may produce dental erosion. Maintaining good general hydration is of course important for the normal functioning of the salivary glands.

The lips should be smeared with cerate or Vaseline.

Oral care of patients with dentures

The daily cleaning of the dentures is carried out with a denture-brush and water. A suitable fluid soap or special denture soaking agents help with the cleaning. Before the dentures are replaced, the oral cavity should also be cleaned (*Figure 10*).

A common cause of denture stomatitis and angular cheilitis is colonisation by yeast in the layer of plaque that forms on the fitting surface of the denture. Antifungal treatment is often needed but proper denture hygiene is important to prevent re-infection.

In order to reduce the risk of stomatitis and denture sore mouth it is

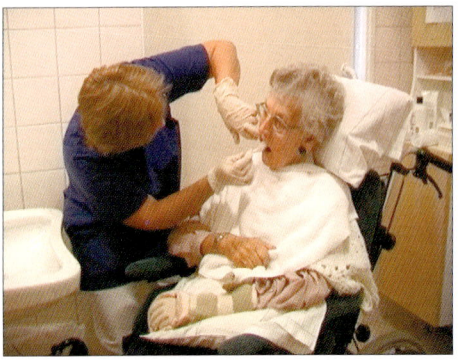

Figure 10
Careful cleaning of the palate.

also recommended that the dentures are removed and kept in fresh water during the night.

Calculus sometimes deposits on a denture. Acetic acid can be used to remove it. The denture is kept in a 6% solution of acetic acid for some hours, then brushed and rinsed in water. If the result is not good enough, the denture should be professionally cleaned.

Dentures that will not be used for a few days or weeks should be kept wet. After a careful cleaning with a brush, the denture is disinfected in chlorhexidine solution 0.2 or 0.1% for 15 minutes. The denture should then be rinsed in water and stored in a suitable way, for example in a closed plastic bag with a wet piece of gauze.

Technical aids in oral self-care for patients with special needs

In order to support the patient to make it possible for him /her to do at least some of the cleaning without assistance, the patient needs technical aids and methodical instruction. This should be provided by a dental hygienist and a physiotherapist and/or an occupational therapist.

Posture

To create the necessary conditions for a person to succeed in cleaning the mouth by themselves, posture is of great importance. Problems caused by high muscle tone and altered motor ability will reduce the control and encourage unwanted movements. For example, the muscle tone will increase when a person with spastic muscles stands up during the oral hygiene procedure. This will lead to stiffer movements, impaired control of balance and a diminished power of concentration. Sitting down in front of the washbasin with a proper arm support and with a mirror at face height will facilitate cleaning of the mouth.

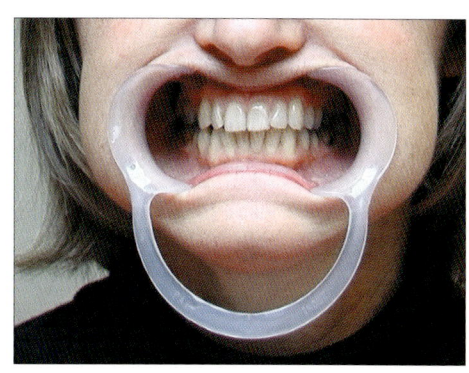

Cheek retractor

For some patients, e.g. with high muscle tone, it is difficult to concentrate on two or more things at the same time, for instance keeping the mouth open and brushing the teeth.

A cheek retractor, common equipment for intraoral photography, will help the person to keep the mouth open without too much effort (*Figure 11*).

Grip aids for toothbrushes

The most common tool for effective mechanical control of dental plaque is a toothbrush. For patients who have impaired muscle function or strength in hands or arms there can be problems. Some examples of grip aids that can compensate for the dysfunction are given below.

It is well-known that the shape of the handle as well as the texture of the material is important for its grip. The market offers different toothbrushes with adequate design for people with a need for enlarged handles. Sometimes the patient's ordinary toothbrush or special brush, like an interdental brush, have to be adapted with a thicker handle. Pieces of foam- or silicone-tubes or any standard plastic- or foam grip handle can be used over the existing handle (*Figure 12*).

There are technical aids that have other functions, but which can be used for a toothbrush too, e.g. holder for spoon or fork attached to the hand by help of Velcro® closing (*Figure 13*).

Double toothbrush

The purpose of this construction of toothbrush is to brush all surfaces of the teeth at the same time (*Figure 14*). This technique is very easy to carry out. The double toothbrush is appreciated as an aid for persons who need help as well as for nurses carrying out the cleaning.

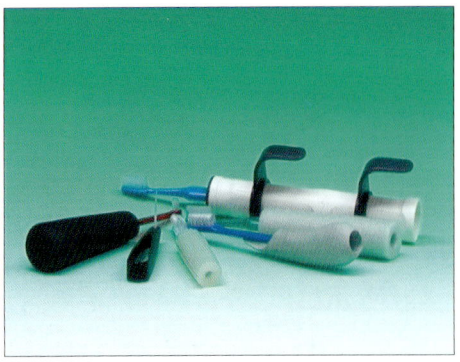

Figure 12
Toothbrushes with enlarged grips.

Figure 13
A holder made of nylon fabric with a pocket for spoon or fork can also be used for a toothbrush.

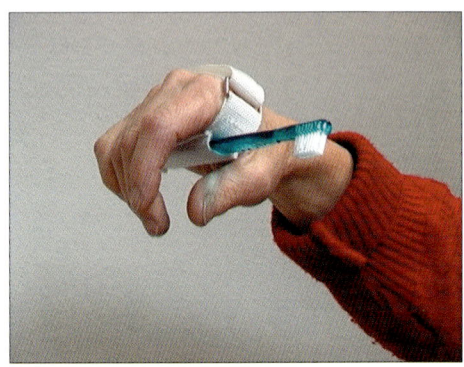

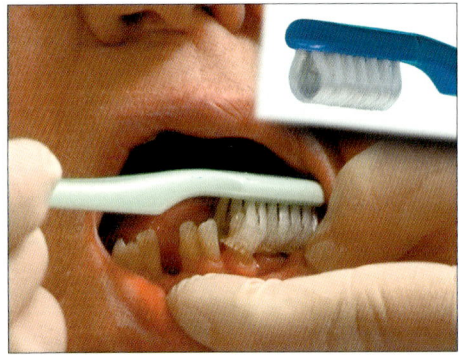

Figure 14
A special design of double toothbrush with opposing, curved bristles cleaning along lingual and buccal gumline simultaneously. One advantage is that there is a very little risk of hurting the mucous membranes or initiating the vomiting-reflex when using this brush.

Battery operated toothbrush

A battery operated brush is a great help as its action compensates for the loss of the skilled manipulation required when using an ordinary toothbrush. As an example, patients with rheumatoid arthritis or muscle diseases often do not have the strength to brush. The powered toothbrush should be light and easy to handle (*Figure 15*).

A battery operated toothbrush is also an excellent tool for patients with difficulties in carrying out isolated hand-movements. These patients often have problems in directing the toothbrush in the oral cavity. The

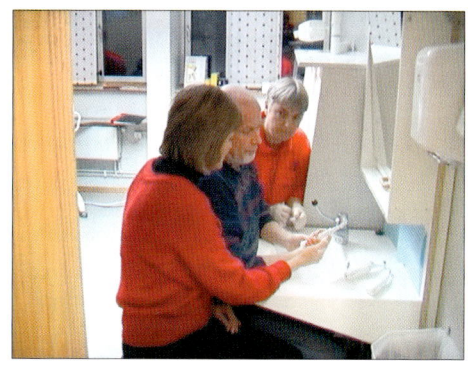

Figure 15

A dental hygienist and an occupational therapist have chosen and adjusted a battery operated toothbrush for a person with weak strength and mobility in arms and hands.

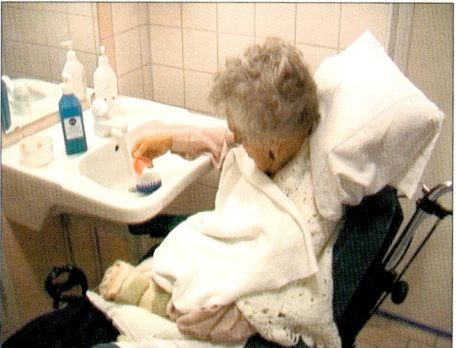

Figure 16

A hemiplegic patient using her only functioning hand to keep the denture and brush it against a denture-brush fixed in the washbasin by a rubber cup.

handle must give a stable grip and its shape should enable the patient to feel how to manipulate the brush in the mouth adequately during cleaning. It is also necessary to instruct in the brushing-technique, step by step.

Another quality of the powered toothbrush that is of great value for some people, is the vibration that stimulates feeling and movements within the mouth.

Denture toothbrush for patients with one-hand function

A patient with function in only one hand cannot hold the denture and brush it at the same time, unless there is an adequate aid as for instance a brush attached to the washbasin (*Figure 16*).

Conclusion

Co-operation between the patient, the dental team, the nursing staff and the patients attendant enables:
- prevention of unnecessary suffering caused by oral diseases
- a better quality of life
- a feeling of comfort
- the possibility of enjoying meals.

Chapter 5

Diet and Nutrition for People with Impairments

Paula Moynihan

Introduction

People with physical and neurological impairments often require dietary modifications as part of their management and this may predispose to increased risk of dental caries. Dental disease increases the burden of ill health, and dental pain in a patient who cannot communicate will exacerbate negative behaviour and feeding difficulties. The aim of this chapter is to provide background information on the feeding problems and dietary management of people with impairments, including neurological dysfunction (cerebral palsy, Down syndrome), inborn errors of metabolism that result in neurological damage (maple syrup urine disease, phenylketonuria, homocystineuria), and patients with chronic physical disabilities (Muscular Dystrophy, Spina Bifida, Juvenile Idiopathic Arthritis). The dental health problems associated with the nutritional management of these conditions, and the means to minimise these, will be considered.

Feeding difficulties in people with neurological dysfunction

Children and adults with neurological dysfunction, for example cerebral palsy and Down syndrome, may have problems with oromotor development which affects their ability to suck and swallow foods. In severe cases in infants this sometimes necessitates nasogastric or gastrostomy feeding. Efforts to improve oromotor function have not been shown to be successful despite several techniques to improve feeding[1,2]. Swallowing difficulty results in prolonged oral retention of foods, which increases the cariogenic potential of some foods[3]. Patients with poor oromotor function are at risk of aspirating and therefore can only tolerate small volumes of foods. This necessitates eating a 'little and often' a practice which is not conducive to good dental health.

It is difficult to achieve an adequate fluid intake in these patients partly because thin fluids are difficult to manipulate in the mouth when swallowing ability is poor. To help overcome this (and reduce the risk of aspiration) thickeners are often added to fluid components of the diet. Cornflour or arrowroot may be use for this purpose but these require pre-cooking prior to addition to the milk feed or drink, which is time consuming. Proprietary thickeners are available on prescription. Some of these are based on non-starch polysaccharide gums that are calorie-free and non-cariogenic; however, many contain maltodextrins (glucose polymers) which are potentially cariogenic[4,5]. Thickening agents that contain maltodextrins are sometimes recommended in preference to gum based thickeners because of the extra energy they provide. An alternative method used to achieve adequate fluid intake is to feed high water content foods in-between meals. Foods recommended for this purpose include fruit-based baby foods, pureed fruit, thick yogurts, fromage frais, ice cream and ice lollies – all of which contain cariogenic sugars and many that are acid. Chewing difficulties, which are often experienced[6], lead to the avoidance of many whole fruits, vegetables and meats. Many foods may have to be liquidised which increases the 'free sugars' (non-milk extrinsic sugars) content of the diet and therefore the cariogenic potential. In some cases it may take up to five years of weaning before semi-solid foods are accepted[7]. Gastrooesophageal reflux is common in severely retarded patients[8] and decreases the oral pH – this, and anticonvulsant-induced vomiting, carry the risk of dental erosion. Reduced saliva production may also be present in some patients – another factor that will increase their caries risk. The feeding difficulties associated with neurological dysfunction are summarised in *Table 1*.

Table 1. Feeding difficulties in people with neurological dysfunction

- Suck-swallow incoordination
- Chewing difficulties
- Swallowing difficulties (retention of food in the oral cavity, aspiration)
- Oral hypersensitivity
- Gastroesophageal reflux
- Reduced appetite (illness, oral hypersensitivity, anticonvulsant therapy)

Failure to Thrive (FTT) and low weight for height

Energy intakes of people with neurological dysfunction are often inadequate. Low energy intake is often the result of feeding difficulties coupled with oral hypersensitivity – which may lead to refusal of food. Anticonvulsant therapy also reduces the appetite. In addition, a patient with Down syndrome or cerebral palsy is prone to infections and ill health, which reduce appetite and increase nutritional requirements when healthy. It is therefore not surprising that Failure to Thrive (FTT) and low body weight have frequently been reported in children with neurological dysfunction[7,9–11]. Stunting of growth is the chronic effect of undernutrition. FTT is characterised by a downward trend in the weight gain trajectory. A weight that is persistently two major centiles below the height centile is considered to be FTT[12].

An energy intake of 1.5 – 2.0 times the normal requirement is recommended for children who are failing to thrive. This is difficult to achieve in the patient with neurological dysfunction and necessitates several dietary practices, which conflict with usual advice for diet and dental health. The diet must be composed of energy dense foods high in fat and/or sugar, such as full-cream milk, cheese, bread spread thickly with butter, cakes, chocolate, biscuits. Feeding difficulties and the time involved in feeding (especially if behavioural problems exist) necessitate small frequent meals. It has been reported that feeding a child with cerebral palsy may take up 4–6 hours each day[13].

It is sometimes not possible to meet the energy requirements with a normal diet and foods are often fortified with glucose polymer powders to increase the energy density of the diet. Glucose polymers may be added to drinks, soup, custards, gravy, mashed potato, stew, porridge, and desserts. The tendency to retain foods in the mouth will result in increased time available for salivary amylase to hydrolyse glucose polymers to glucose, maltose and short chain oligosaccharides. Therefore foods which have been fortified with glucose polymers which also tend to be held in the mouth carry a caries risk.

Nutritional supplements (fruit based drinks or milk-based drinks) may be prescribed to increase the nutrient density of the diet. It is recommended that these be taken between meals so that they supplement, rather than replace, usual food intake. Nutritional supplements vary in composition: some are energy supplements composed of carbohydrate (sugars and glucose polymers) with or without fat emulsions, and some have a protein component. However, most nutritional supplements contain both sugars and glucose polymers. Many of these drinks come in Tetrapaks with a drinking straw provided.

Infants with inadequate growth may be recommended 'follow on formula' to increase the energy density of the diet. This is an energy-enriched formula that has added glucose polymers. For a normal child it is recommended that follow-on formula is given in a cup, to reduce the risk of nursing bottle caries, however, this may not be possible in the infant with impairments. Glucose polymers may be added to normal formula milk as an alternative to follow-on formulas. For healthy children, bottle-feeding sugar-containing foods and drinks at bed-time is a practice which is discouraged, for dental health reasons. However, for a child that has a low weight or is failing to thrive, a bed-time feed can provide an important opportunity to increase the child's energy intake and therefore, in some cases, it may not be appropriate to discourage this practice. The dietary practices, of patients with neuro-

Table 2. Dietary practices of patients with neurological dysfunction, which may cause dental health problems

- Increased oral retention of foods
- Use of thickening agents containing maltodextrins
- Energy dense diet high in sugars and glucose polymers
- Small and frequent meals
- Gastroesophageal reflux and vomiting
- Sugars and glucose polymers near bedtime
- Follow-on formula in bottles (or glucose polymer-containing formula)
- Follow on formula at bedtime (or glucose-polymer-containing formula)
- Extended period of bottle feeding
- Liquidised foods (containing 'free sugars'/non-milk extrinsic sugars)

logical dysfunctions, which increase the risk of dental caries and dental erosion are summarised in *Table 2*.

The use of glucose polymers

Glucose polymers (glucose syrups and maltodextrins) are derived from starch and are comprised of chains of 3–20 glucose units along with glucose and maltose. Maltodextrins are relatively more complex in structure than glucose syrups, however, both can be broken down by salivary amylase to mono and di- saccharides. The limited information on the dental health effects of these carbohydrates suggest that both are potentially cariogenic[4,5]. The oral retention time and the mode of consumption of foods and drinks containing glucose polymers are important.

Advice to minimise dental diseases in patients with neurological dysfunctions

For the patient with neurological impairments, preventive dentistry must largely focus on oral hygiene, exposure to appropriate fluoride levels and regular dental attendance. However, there are some dietary measures which may be employed to safeguard the dentition. How feasible these measures are depends on the circumstances of each individual case and advice should be tailored and monitored to suit each patient. Suggested dietary recommendations for minimising caries are presented in *Table 3*.

Inborn errors of metabolism which cause neurological dysfunction

Maple syrup urine disease

Maple syrup urine disease (MSUD) is caused by a deficiency of the enzyme branched-chain ketoacid dehydrogenase which results in accumulation of branched chain amino acids (BCAA) and their ketoacids.

Table 3. Possible recommendations for dietary practices to mimimise caries in patients with impairments

1) If a bed-time feed or snack/meal is necessary, one which is low in sugars can be negotiated e.g. bread and butter or cheese for children who tolerate solid foods or full-fat milk for any child.

2) If a thickening agent is used one which does not contain maltodextrins may be recommended unless it is essential to have a maltodextrin-containing thickener for the provision of calories.

3) Wherever possible children should be weaned onto a cup or encouraged to drink from a straw – the feasibility of this depends of the degree of impairment.

4) It is best if glucose polymers are only added to foods that are cleared relatively quickly from the mouth – e.g. drinks. It must be recognised that this may not be possible if a child is failing to thrive

This causes irreversible neurological impairment. A diet low in leucine and other BCAA is essential to minimise neurological impairment[14,15].

Phenylketonuria (PKU) is an inborn error of amino acid metabolism that results in failure to metabolise phenylalanine. Failure to diagnose this condition at birth results in severe neurological impairment. The dietary management is a low phenylalanine diet.

Homocystinuria is another inborn error in which plasma levels of homocystine are raised and methionine is not metabolised properly. Clinical manifestations include skeletal abnormalities and neurological complications that develop in later childhood[16].

In all conditions that involve failure to metabolise a certain amino acid, the patient follows a very low protein diet, high in sugar and fat, and receive their protein as an amino acid supplement and low biological value exchanges. The diet is based on providing the minimum amount of the 'toxic' amino acid (i.e. BCAA, phenylalanine, methionine) that is required for growth. This is provided from foods of low biological value protein. Other essential amino acids are provided as a supplement drink. Non-protein high-energy foods are promoted, as an inadequate energy intake will result in protein catabolism and an increase in plasma concentrations of the 'toxic' amino acid or its metabolites. Sugar-rich foods and high-fat foods that are low in protein are therefore encouraged and include sugar, preserves, boiled sweets, margarine and oils. Specially manufactured low protein foods are available on prescription and include bread, biscuits (sweet and savoury) and pasta. Low protein foods are made from highly refined flour and have a tendency to stick to the teeth, which is likely to increase the cariogenic potential of these products. To ensure an adequate energy intake, products containing glucose polymers, sucrose and fat emulsions (e.g. chocolate substitute and energy fortifying powders) are available on prescription.

The main dental health concerns for all these conditions is the frequent and high intake of sugar and glucose polymers. Patients with

PKU must also avoid all foods and drinks containing the non-sugar sweetener aspartame (Canderell, Nutra-Sweet) as it is made from phenylalanine.

Chronic physical impairment

Physical impairments that predispose to nutritional problems include muscular dystrophy, spina bifida and juvenile idiopathic arthritis. The nutritional problems associated with chronic physical impairment include overweight, underweight and poor growth and constipation.

Immobility reduces the energy requirement in muscular dystrophy and spina bifida and this often results in weight gain. Parents often give high-energy snacks and sweets as sympathy rewards and this exacerbates the problem. Overweight children and adults with chronic physical impairments should have their intake of sweet-fat-rich and fat rich foods restricted – this should not conflict with advice for dental health.

Children with juvenile idiopathic arthritis (JIA) often exhibit growth retardation and protein energy malnutrition[17,18] and are shorter than healthy children. Possible factors contributing to nutritional impairment include anorexia, inappropriate 'alternative' diets, increased energy requirements during periods of active disease, persistent disease activity[17,19,20], and mechanical feeding difficulties. This may necessitate the provision of an energy dense diet that may be high in cariogenic carbohydrates. Frequent provision of sweets as treats has been reported in children with chronic idiopathic arthritis[21]. Patients with JIA may experience pain in the temporomandibular joint which predisposes to chewing difficulties and patients may also have pain in their hands and difficulty using cutlery. The increase nutritional requirements and feeding difficulties experienced by some children with JIA may place them at increase risk of dental caries and increased levels of dental caries has been reported in this group[22]. Increasing awareness of the dental health risk of children with JIA, focusing on stringent oral hygiene measures and reducing the frequency of intake of sugar-containing foods are important preventive strategies for these patients.

In conclusion, the dietary management and nutritional problems of patients with neurological, metabolic or physical impairments may place them at increased risk of dental caries and/or dental erosion. To minimise the risk of these oral diseases it is important that dental health professionals appreciate where the compromise between diet for growth and disease management and diet for dental health lies, so that the patient receives sound, consistent dietary messages from all health professionals. Good, professional relationships between dietitians, medical practitioners, paediatricians and dental health professionals are essential for this purpose.

References

1. Bax M. Eating is important. *Dev Med Child Neurol* 1989; **31:** 285–286.
2. Matisen B. Oral-motor dysfunction and failure to thrive among inner-city infants. *Dev Med Child Neurol* 1989; **31:** 293–302.
3. Pollard M A. Potential cariogenicity of starches and fruits as assessed by the plaque sampling method and an intraoral cariogenicity test. *Caries Res* 1996; **29:** 68–74.
4. Moynihan P J, Gould M E L, Huntley N, Thorman S. Effect of glucose polymers in water, milk and a milk substitute on plaque pH in vitro. *Int J Paed Dent* 1996; **6:** 19–24.
5. Grenby T H, Mistry M. Potential cariogenicity of glucose syrups and maltodextrins. *Caries Res* 1996; **30:** 289.
6. Dyke D V. *Problems in Feeding.* New York: Springer-Verlag; 1990.
7. Webb Y. Feeding and nutritional problems of physically and mentally handicapped children in Britain: a report. *J Hum Nutr* 1980; **34:** 241–285.
8. Sondheimer J M, Morris B A. Gastroesophageal reflux among severely retarded children. *J Pediat* 1979; **94:** 710–714.
9. Karle I P. Nutritional status of cerebral palsied children. *J Am Dietet Assoc* 1961; **38:** 22–26.
10. Krick J, Duyne M V. The relationship between oral-motor involvement and growth: a pilot study in paediatric population with cerebral palsy. *J Am Dietet Assoc* 1984; **84 (5):** 555–559.
11. Thommessen M, Heiberg A, Kase B F, Larsen S, Riis G. Feeding problems, height and weight in different groups of disabled children. *Acta Paediatr Scand* 1991; **80:** 527–533.
12. White F. *Failure to thrive.* Oxford: Blackwell Scientific Publications, 1994.
13. Jones A M. Overcoming the feeding problems of the mentally and physically handicapped. *J Hum Nutr* 1978; **32:** 359–367.
14. Hilliges C, Awuszus D, Wendel U. Intellectual performance of children with maple syrup urine disease. *Eur J Paed* 1993; **152:** 144–147.
15. Nord A, Doornick W, Greene C. Developmental profile of patients with maple syrup urine disease. *J Inher Metab Dis* 1991; **14:** 881–889.
16. Mudd S H, Levy H L, Skovby R. *Disorders of trans-sulfuration.* New York: McGraw-Hill, 1989.
17. Johansson U, Portinsson S, Akesson A, Svantesson H, Ockerman P A, Akesson B. Nutritional status in girls with juvenile chronic arthritis. *Hum Nutr Clin Nutr* 1986; **40C:** 57–67.
18. Henderson C J, Lovell D J. Assessment of protein-energy malnutrition in children and adolescents with juvenile rheumatoid arthritis. *Arthr Care Res* 1989; **2:** 108–113.
19. Miller M L, Chacko J A, Young E A. Dietary deficiencies in children with juvenile rheumatoid arthritis. *Arthr Care Res* 1989; **2:** 22–24.
20. Haugen M A, Hoyeraal H M, Larsen S, MGilboe I, Trygg K. Nutrient intake and nutritional status in children with juvenile chronic arthritis. *Rheumatology* 1992; **21:** 165–170.
21. Moynihan P J, Welbury R, Foster H, Kerber M, Thomason J M. Is juvenile idiopathic arthritis associated with dietary practices, which increase the risk of dental caries? In: *EULAR, 1999.* Glasgow, 1999.
22. Fitzgerald J, Welbury R R, Foster H E, Stephenson S, Marshall N, Wallis J, et al. The oral health in children and young adults with juvenile idiopathic arthritis in the North of England. In: *EULAR, 1999.* Glasgow, 1999.

Chapter 6

General Health Assessment

Daniel Jolly

Introduction

Oral health care has become a greater priority as people live longer with serious medical conditions and disabilities. In addition, they require more comprehensive dental treatment. As a result dental (oral health) care is becoming an increasingly integrated part of overall medical care.

Therefore, we are now faced with more serious decisions requiring the use of our cognitive resources to decide how oral health care affects not only an individual's quality of life, but also their quantity of life. Oral health care treatment plans must therefore be optimised and interdisciplinary. These concepts have been described in more detail in recent publications[1-9].

Definitions

A medically compromised dental patient is one who has a general health condition, physical, mental, and/or emotional who must alter their activities from "normal" and who requires some kind of modification in the usual pattern of receiving oral health care.

The scope of compromising medical conditions and disabilities can vary widely. It might be an individual with a mild heart murmur who requires only pre-treatment antibiotics. It could be an individual with multiple organ system failure who can only be treated in a hospital environment. It can also include patients who require additional time for dental treatment because of physical, communicative, and/or cognitive disabilities.

A medically compromising condition or impairment can be manifested in the same fashion as a physical, mental, or developmental disability. It creates a lifestyle for an individual which limits the "normal" Activities of Daily Living (ADLs). Identification of the medical conditions in these patients is critical. Inappropriate identification, through improper history taking and interpretation, can create ineffective, or even detrimental, oral health care treatment.

Information gathering

To properly identify a patient's medical condition, an adequate medical history must be taken. In many cases, the patient does not interpret systemic illnesses, signs, symptoms, medications, etc. as relevant to the practice of dentistry. As a result, a simple question and answer form completed by the patient may not reveal relevant medical information. The dentist must therefore conduct a verbal (or other appropriate) interview of the patient, family member, carer, nurse, etc.

A summary of the importance of medical history and physical evaluation is provided by Morgan L. Allison, DDS. He has stated that "When you listen, hear; when you look, see; when you touch, feel"[10]. In other words, the process of obtaining a medical history is an active and interactive action or set of actions. After information is gathered from the patient or other appropriate sources, it can be analysed and an appropriate reaction (treatment plan) can be developed. Numerous other authors and clinicians had written on this topic as well[11-14].

First, when you gather a medical history, a written guideline (questionnaire) can be used to provide a baseline. Next, let the patient talk to you and then listen closely Many times a patient will diagnose himself or herself in this manner. After the patient has provided written and verbal information, the dentist must ask appropriate questions. Appropriate questions are open ended and require the patient to synthesise an answer.

The dentist, after reviewing the information provided can then ask a question such as "Tell me about how it is that you get out of breath so easily". Please refer to *Table 1* for a more complete summary of the pertinent topics on which to question a patient.

A developmental history must always be included. This should define the nature of the illness or disability and how that person has developed and functioned in his or her social, family, work or educational setting. Behavioural patterns must be assessed to determine functional capacity of the individual to receive treatment or to provide (or be provided with) oral health care in the daily setting.

The patient (or the patient's carer) must be questioned about family and social history. Certain medical conditions such as cardiac disease and cancer have strong familial inheritance patterns. Certain disabilities are known to have associated medical conditions such as congenital heart disease and Down syndrome or cerebral palsy and convulsions.

Medication history is critical to properly assess. Many patients are unaware of their actual "drug" usage. Prescribed drugs are often not remembered specifically by the patient. Drugs, medications or herbal remedies and products available without a prescription are often not considered significant but could interact negatively with prescribed

Table 1. Medical history topic questions

Identification
- name, age, race, sex (may also include name of referring physician and name of informant.)

CC: (Chief complaint)
- stated in patient's own words if possible

HPI: (History of Present Illness HOPI or HPI)
- course of present illness; how and when it began
- pertinent positive and negative review of systems
- risk factors
- diagnostic tests done
- related illnesses

PMH: (Past Medical History)
- hospital admissions
- prior surgery
- medical condition

FHx: (Family History)
- Lives at home, with spouse, children, institution...
- Medical problems in any blood relative (cancer, TB, allergy, asthma, cardiovascular disease, renal disease, ulcers, diabetes, haemophilia)

SHx: (Social History)
- Tobacco
- Alcohol use and abuse
- present and past employment
- exposure to environmental agents
- hobbies
- water supply
- sleep and play habits (paediatric)
- Drug use and abuse
- marital status
- support
- religion, beliefs
- living conditions
- travel abroad

ROS: (Review of Systems)

General:	Weight change, weakness, fatigue, fever, chills, sweats
Skin:	rashes, pruritus, lesions
Head:	trauma, headache, tenderness
Eyes:	vision, changes in visual field, glasses, last prescription change, photophobia, blurring, diplopia, spots, inflammation, discharge
Ears:	hearing changes, tinnitus, pain, discharge, vertigo
Nose:	sinus problems, bleeding, obstruction, polyps
Throat:	teeth, tongue, gums, dentures, lesions, hoarseness, tonsils, palate, pharynx
Respiratory:	chest pain, wheezing, dyspnoea, cough, sputum, amount and colour, haemoptysis
Cardiovascular:	blood pressure, pulse, chest pain, dyspnoea, rheumatic fever, murmurs, orthopnea, number of pillows at night, cyanosis, oedema, claudication
Gastrointestinal:	appetite, dysphagia, nausea, vomiting, haematemesis, indigestion, pain, diarrhoea, constipation, melaena, bloating, anal discomfort, haemorrhoids, stool shape and colour, jaundice
Genitourinary:	frequency, urgency, dysuria, haematuria, nocturia, incontinence, venereal disease, discharge, sterility, impotence
Gynaecological:	Gravida/para/abortion (G3,P2,A1), last menstrual period (LMP), frequency, duration, flow, dysmennorhea, spotting, menopause, contraception, last pelvic and pap smear,
Endocrine:	polyuria, polydypsia, polyphagia, temperature intolerance, thyroid difficulties, glycosuria, hormone therapy
Musculoskeletal:	arthritis, trauma, swelling
Haematology:	anaemia, bleeding tendency, easy bruising, lymphadenopathy
Neuropsychiatric:	syncope, seizures, weakness, coordination, sensations, memory, mood, sleep pattern, emotional disturbances, drug or alcohol abuse

medications. This would include aspirin, antacids, vitamins, cold medications, etc. A patient must also be asked about other "drugs, pills, elixirs, liquids, syrups, tablets, vitamins, compounds, etc." A drug allergy history needs to be investigated and the patient's reaction needs to be classified as an allergic reaction or an intolerance.

In summary, information gathering should take the form of a structured interview. Look for the signs and symptoms associated with the conditions(s) with which the patient presents. Enquire about family and social history such as inherited diseases like cardiovascular, respiratory, cancer, diabetes, etc.

Collect details of the patient history within the context of the patient, such as their daily activities and overall functions, available support and identify physicians with whom the dentist should liaise.

Examination

Next, the dentist must assess and record vital signs (blood pressure, pulse, respiration, and temperature).

Evaluation of the heart must include questions about rheumatic fever, heart attacks, chest pain, and breathlessness for example. Assessment can be aided by observing for swollen extremities and/or cyanosis in the patient's skin. Congestive heart failure, and therefore valvular disease, can be identified by breathlessness on exertion or fluid accumulation in the extremities. Chest pain can be indicative of coronary artery disease and/or valvular disease. Conditions which include scoliosis and kyphosis predispose to altered cardiac and respiratory function (*Figure 1*). Tolerance for oral health care treatment is thereby affected and must be accurately assessed.

The respiratory system must be evaluated as well. Again, breathlessness, during rest, exertion, sleep, etc. should be investigated.

Figure 1

Skeletal comparison of a normal spine and scoliosis

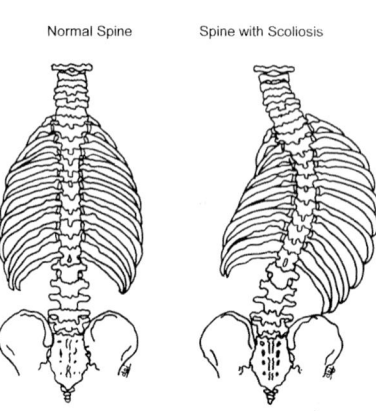

Normal Spine Spine with Scoliosis

Environmental allergies and the related respiratory difficulties must be differentiated from emphysema, asthma, pneumonia, or neoplasia. Physical impairments may have an impact on respiratory function.

The function of the liver needs to be assessed by inquiries addressing bleeding problems, jaundice, history of hepatitis, etc. Renal function must also be evaluated since drug metabolism is critical in the routine management of the dental patient. Endocrine disorders such as diabetes and thyroid disease can be readily investigated via the history.

The patient with endocrine disorders can potentially develop life threatening problems during dental treatment. The diabetic patient could become hypoglycaemic during a dental appointment because of too little food intake and irregular or too much insulin administration. Thyroid patients, particularly those with hyperthyroidism can react to vasoconstrictors in dental anaesthetics with significantly elevated blood pressure. Fits and convulsions are a significant barrier to routine oral health care. A fit during dental treatment can lead to aspiration of dental materials or instruments. Removable prostheses, portions of fractured porcelain from a fixed prosthesis or even fractured teeth and simple restorations can be aspirated. Maintaining a stress-free clinical environment or reducing stress with agents such as diazepam or nitrous oxide can be useful preventive actions.

An additional component of obtaining and evaluating a medical history is medical consultation. Requesting appropriate information from a patient's physician(s) is often a necessary activity. Requests for physician's opinion should always be provided in the context of the necessary dental treatment. Usually, the dentist can properly evaluate a patient and decide on the appropriate medical management considerations. The dentist will, more often than not, only require the physician to provide confirmation of the plan, assist in the management, or occasionally add previously unknown information to the patient history.

One additional aspect of the evaluation of the medical history is the consideration of all the other "non-medical" factors present in a patient's life. These are outlined more completely in *Table 2*.

Risk assessment

The evaluation process will conclude with the designation of the patient as meeting the medical risk criteria according to the American Association of Anesthesiologists. An additional assessment tool is the Prognosis and Assessment of Risk (PARS) Scale. This evaluation scale is outlined in *Tables 3 and 4*. It can function in conjunction with the more well known Frankl and American Society of Anesthesiology Scales[15–16] for patient care evaluation. This scale can be useful in educating the

Table 2. Dental risk assessment and prognosis evaluation scale

---

Modification Considerations

All the PARS categories are modified by an individual evaluation of the patient aspects itemised in the section on Risk Assessment. These general categories include:

1. *Medical and Physical status*: What complicating medical conditions exist? This is a large item of consideration which will be clarified by other chapters of this publication.

2. *Oral Hygiene*: What are the patient's abilities and level of interest in oral health as evidenced by the current condition and past dental history.

3. *Psychological needs*: What are the aesthetic and functional factors which would improve the individual's self image and willingness to function in society, at work at school and with peers.

4. *Functional ability*: What is the level of function in the community in which the patient lives

5. *Mental status*: What is the level of understanding and communication of the patient?

6. *Social status*: What is the patient's work and school environment?

7. *Family status*: What is the patient's home and living environment, availability and level of understanding of caregivers?

8. *Physical limitations*: What ability does the patient have to provide their own oral hygiene care?

9. *Accessibility issues*: Can the patient receive dental treatment in the dental surgery environment, physically enter the office and move safely around in the office; does the patient have a way to travel to the office for frequent, occasional, annual or only emergency visits?

10. *Financial issues:* Can the patient afford the recommended treatment or what alternatives and compromises are feasible for the individual?

11. *Communication needs:* Can the patient understand instructions, require an interpreter or communicate his or her concerns directly to the dental team in an appropriate fashion?

12. *Appropriate behaviour management* needs to be planned: What medications, restraints, informed consent, extra time allowance, hospitalisation, etc. need to be considered?

13. *Consent:* Is the patient able to provide his or her own consent or is another individual, group of individuals, agency or court responsible?

---

young dental professional in appropriate initial considerations in treatment planning for the medically compromised patient.

Category I: A healthy and co-operative patient who requires no special modifications to receive dental care. Dental treatment planning would not have to consider any medical implications. Acute and chronic dental disease can be managed in a routine manner. The ASA scale that correlates with this category is ASA-I and is designated as a healthy person.

Category II: A person with a medical condition or disability who requires some non-routine considerations to receive dental care. Dental treatment should focus on elimination of acute infection prior to a medical or surgical procedure. Acute disease, such as a periapical abscess, generally should be treated by extraction. Chronic disease which can be maintained in control can be treated after the medical or surgical treatment. Prosthetic heart valve patients are an example. A relatively co-operative person, perhaps one with mild mental retarda-

Table 3. Prognosis and assessment of risk scale (PARS)

Category descriptions	Type & timing of treatment							
	Before[1]					After[2]		
	R[3]	N[4]	S[5]	A[6]	M[7]	R[3]	C[8]	L[9]
Category I Healthy patient No special modifications	X					X		
Category II Medical condition who requires some non-routine considerations to receive dental care and co-operative patient with diminished mental and physical function but the ability to perform or permit adequate oral hygiene procedures on a daily basis. This category might include the patient with mild mental retardation but who is co-operative for most dental care.		X				X		
Category III Medical condition with significant life-long implications and requires significant modifications in dental treatment planning. Includes the patient with management requirements for behavioural purposes that includes sedation and other mild anaesthesia techniques and who can not perform daily adequate oral hygiene routinely without significant assistance. This would include the moderately unco-operative dental patient with cerebral palsy, neuromuscular disorders or more severe mental deficits that is uncooperative and could not maintain or permit someone else to maintain complicated oral appliances and restorations			X				X	
Category IV Medical condition which necessitates major modifications in dental treatment planning. Includes patients requiring deep sedation and general anaesthesia for behaviour control and the patient who permits minimal oral hygiene care.				X				X
Category V Serious medical condition which necessitates only limited care to eliminate serious acute oral disease. Includes the combative patient with no ability to provide oral hygiene care.					X	Does not apply		

Footnotes: Please refer to *Table 4*

tion, who can provide his or her basic oral care (or permit it to be provided) would fit this category. This correlates to the ASA II designation which includes mild controlled systemic disease such as well controlled hypertension and well controlled diabetes.

Category III: A person with a medical condition which has significant lifelong implications for the patient. Dental care should focus on elimination of acute infection and removal of chronic problems and disease states prior to the medical or surgical procedure. Extractions would be indicated for teeth with periapical abscesses or for teeth with moderate to severe periodontal disease. Organ transplant patients are prime examples of this category. People with disabilities who require treatment under some forms of sedation might fit this category. These

Table 4. Dental risk assessment and prognosis evaluation scale

Type and timing of treatment (explanation of footnotes from Table 3)

1. *Before:* Types of treatment considerations prior to the planned medical or surgical therapy

2. *After:* Types of treatment considerations after completion of medical or surgical therapy.

3. *Routine:* No alterations prior to or following medical or surgical therapy except those which are routinely made secondary to "normal" treatment planning and patient specific considerations. Some medical management preparation may be required.

4. *Non-routine:* Extract teeth with periapical lesions, abscesses, furcations more than Grade II, mobility more than Grade II, and those with a potential for endodontic complications (large caries, etc.). Prophy prior to therapy. Minor medical management preparation required. Oral hygiene history and potential and other patient factors can modify treatment plan significantly.

5. *Significant:* Extract teeth with periapical lesions, abscesses, furcations of Grade II or more, mobility of Grade II or more, impacted third molars, and those with a potential for endodontic complications. Prophy prior to therapy. Significant medical management preparation required. Modifying factors will usually not significantly modify treatment plan.

6. *Aggressive:* Extract impacted teeth and those with abscesses, large caries, periapical pathology, periodontal disease, and any potential for infectious and/or septic complications. Prophy of remaining teeth prior to therapy. Significant medical management preparation may be required. Modifying factors will usually not modify treatment plan at all.

7. *Minimal:* Manage only acute disease to prevent pain and infection with palliative procedures.

8. *Conservative:* Routine dental care generally possible. Evaluate carefully if extensive rehabilitative oral care is planned with fixed prosthetics. Avoid implants or procedures which would potentially exacerbate immunosupressed individuals. Most surgical procedures are generally not contraindicated. Appropriate medical management preparation needs to be considered.

9. *Limited:* Manage only acute disease, Fixed and removable prosthetic rehabilitation may be limited. Surgical procedures exposing bone may require extensive preparation (e.g. hyperbaric oxygen treatments for radiation therapy patients). Will require extensive medical management preparation. Extensive medical management preparation.

people would be able to maintain a natural dentition in fair repair with assistance but not be able to manage complex prosthodontic devices or maintain periodontal surgical sites in a clean and healthy state. This category correlates to ASA III which is defined as severe disease that is not incapacitating. This ASA category includes such conditions as poorly controlled convulsions.

Category IV: A person with a medical condition which necessitates major modifications in dental treatment planning. Removal of acute and chronic oral disease prior to medical, surgical, or radiological treatment is imperative. All future potential oral disease should be minimised or eliminated prior to the medical therapy. Teeth presenting with large carious cavities and moderate periodontal disease should be extracted. These extractions should be performed even if the condition is one which would be readily treatable in the Category I, II, or III patient. For example, patients with poor oral hygiene, extensive but restorable dental caries, and localised moderate periodontal disease who are to receive radiation therapy to the head and neck should have all teeth with questionable prognosis removed before treatment. People with disabilities who can be treated only under general anaesthesia and permit little oral hygiene to be accomplished for them would also fit this category. The related ASA IV category would include incapacitating systemic disease such as congestive heart failure.

Category V: A person for whom no dental treatment would be indicated except to control acute and chronic infection and establish basic oral function as necessary. A terminally ill patient with a very short life expectancy might be an example of this category. This includes people with impairments who do not permit oral hygiene care.

Modifications: All the categories are modified by an individual evaluation of the categories itemised in *Table 2*. If a patient who generally received a Category III ranking, but the individual evaluation of the modifications listed in *Table 2* were favourable for the patient, that individual might be rated a Category II patient for treatment planning purposes.

These general categories include:

- oral hygiene abilities,
- level of interest in oral health as evidenced by the current condition and past dental history
- urgency of the medical condition
- patient desires
- emotional factors such as self-image,
- level of function in the community in which the patient lives
- other individual factors.

Summary

Medical and dental interdisciplinary co-operation is critical in appropriate assessment of the medical history and the subsequent management of the medically compromised dental patient. This interdisciplinary interactive co-operation must extend beyond the physician and include the patient, family, caregivers, therapists, and anyone else involved in the life of the particular individual.

The critical activity on the part of the dentist in managing the physically, medically, mentally and/or emotionally compromised dental patient is the cognitive skill ability. If properly accomplished, the cognitive skills will permit appropriate use of the proper technique and behavioural skills. Appropriate oral health care can contribute significantly to a person's quantity and quality of life.

It must be remembered that optimum care may not be ideal and will be influenced by the patient and situation specific circumstances. When this approach to treatment is followed in the relevant interdisciplinary fashion, the patient will benefit and an individual's quantity and quality of life should benefit.

Dental care for the patient with medically compromising conditions and disabilities can be difficult and infinitely challenging, but ultimately rewarding. Not only do patients benefit, but so does the oral health care provider, health care professions as a whole, and Society. The measure of a success of a society is the measure of the degree to which that society takes care of those of its members who can not take care of themselves. Dental care for the person with medical disabilities is just such an example.

References

1. Shampaine G S. Patient Assessment and Preventive Measures for Medical Emergencies in the Dental Office. *Dent Clin N Am* 1999; **43**: 383–400.
2. Emery R W, Guttenberg S A. Management Priorities for Medical Emergencies in the Dental Office. *Dent Clin N Am* 1999; **43:** 401–420.
3. Glick M. New Guidelines for Prevention, Detection, Evaluation and Treatment of High Blood Pressure. *J Am Dent Assoc* 1998; **129:** 1588–1594.
4. Muzyka B C, Glick M. The Hypertensive Dental Patient. *J Am Dent Assoc* 1997; **128:** 1109–1120.
5. Jolly D. Evaluation of Medical Risk in the Dental Patient. *Anes Prog* 1995; **42:** 90–92.
6. Jolly D. Evaluation of the Medical History. *Anes Prog* 1995; **42:** 84–89.
7. Jolly D. Interpreting the Medical History. *J Calif Dent Assoc* 1995; **23:**19–28.
8. Jolly D. Management of the medically compromised dental patient. *Proceedings of the 11th Congress of the International Association of Dentistry for the Handicapped*. Monduzzi Editore, Bologna, 1992, p 3–10.
9. Jolly D E. Evaluation of the medical history. *Dent Clin N Am* 1994; **38:** 361–308.
10. Allison M L. Personal communication. In: Jolly D E, *Hospital Dental Resident Manual*. The Ohio State University College of Dentistry, 1993; 1–8.
11. Bates B. *A Guide to Physical Examination and History Taking*. 5th ed. St. Louis, C. V. Mosby, 1991; 1–33.
12. Little J W, Falace D A. *Dental Management of the Medically Compromised Patient*. 4th ed. St. Louis, C.V. Mosby, 1993.
13. Lockhart P B. *Oral Medicine and Hospital Practice*. Fourth Edition. Federation of Special Care Organizations in Dentistry, Chicago, 1997; pp 2-4 – 2-15.
14. Rose L F, Kaye D, Steinberg B J. In: Rose L F and Kaye D. *Internal Medicine for Dentistry*. 2. ed. St. Louis, C.V. Mosby, 1990; pp 1–6.
15. American Society of Anesthesiologists. New Classifications of Physical Status. *Anesthesiology* 1963; **24:** 11.
16. Frankl S N, Shiere F R, Fogels H R. Should the parent remain with the child in the dental operatory? *J Dent Child* 1962; **29:** 150–163.

Chapter 7

Assessment for General Anaesthesia

Gary Enever

Introduction

Co-operation is often lacking in patients with severe disability, so care and often examination of their many dental problems[1,2] can only be carried out with the help of sedation or general anaesthesia[3]. However, these patients often have concurrent medical problems which make sedation or anaesthesia potentially hazardous[3-6].

In providing care for these patients, we are often faced with a dilemma. They need their dental care, but at what potential for harm? We then enter into a process of balancing risks and benefits to arrive at what is often a compromise solution. We must be able to assess the potential risks to those we care for, and then deliver the best treatment we can with the resources we have available. With some patients, general anaesthesia is the only means of delivering care, and so we must make it as safe and free from morbidity as possible[7].

We therefore have to consider three aspects of care. Firstly, the resources available to deliver patient care, including staff, equipment and facilities. This allows us to define what care can be safely offered. Secondly, we must look at our patients to assess what potential problems they might have peri-operatively, and decide where their care should be delivered.

Finally, we need to consider the various ways in which assessment can be carried out, to achieve reliable reproducible results with the least inconvenience to our disabled patients and their carers.

Aspects of care:

- Resources available – staff, equipment, facilities and money
- Reliable assessment protocol
- Risk factors peri-operatively

Assessment of resources

Staff

As already stated, patients with disabilities may present anaesthetic staff with considerable difficulties. They must therefore be adequately trained and experienced for the task, which may include the management of difficult airways and complex medical problems, as well as unco-operative patients.

For the same reasons, well trained and experienced nursing staff are extremely important in the smooth handling of people with impairments. They are usually the first point of contact with patient and carers arriving for treatment, and can pick up information which may be vital to the anaesthetist. Secondly, an experienced anaesthetic assistant is very helpful when dealing with difficult children and adults with impairments. Finally, skilled recovery staff are important to ensure a swift and safe return to normal, bearing in mind that 'normal' for that patient may not be the standard data set we assume for non-impaired patients. For example, oxygen saturation in a patient with severe physical impairment and chronic lung disease may be outwith the limits we would regard as 'normal' , although for that particular patient, this is their normal, everyday value.

Without appropriate staffing, the risks are increased to all patients, not only those with disabilities.

Equipment and drugs

The availability of a reasonable selection of modern anaesthetic drugs and equipment will aid the safe delivery of anaesthesia, but will not reduce the need for experienced staff. A skilled anaesthetist can give "safe" anaesthesia with very rudimentary equipment and basic drugs.

Modern drugs undoubtedly reduce morbidity, and allow the minimisation of disruption to patient and carers by reducing the post operative recovery period. The use of short acting drugs such as the intravenous anaesthetic agent propofol, and the inhalational agents isoflurane and sevoflurane have been responsible for this improvement. This is especially true when used with modern muscle relaxant drugs and monitoring, allowing light and easily reversible anaesthesia.

The technique used may for example, involve either a gaseous induction (*Figure 1*) with sevoflurane in oxygen, or intravenous induction with fentanyl 1 microgram per kilogram, propofol 2 milligrams per kilogram, and then vecuronium 0.1 milligram per kilogram for all. Intubation is preferentially nasal, using small soft nasotracheal tubes, and anaesthesia maintained by ventilation with nitrous oxide, oxygen and isoflurane (*Figure 2*). At the end of the dental procedure, patients should be placed on their side, any residual muscle relaxation reversed and 100% oxygen given until spontaneous respiration is established and the patient wakes from anaesthesia. Patients would then be extubated and transferred to the recovery area.

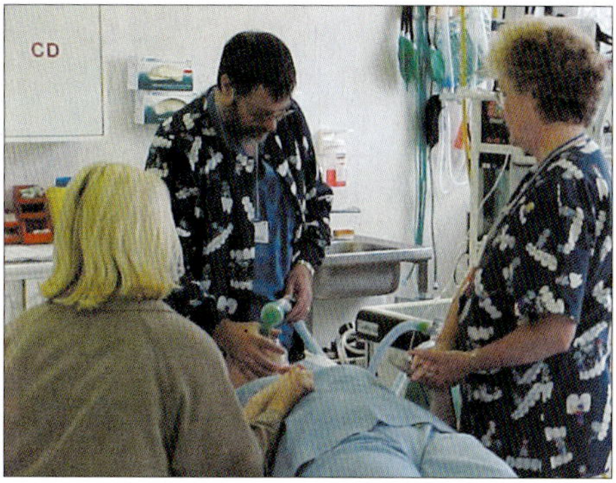

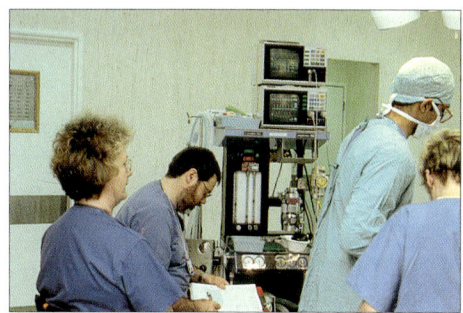

Figure 1
Patient undergoing gaseous induction

Figure 2
Monitoring of anaesthetised patient in the dental theatre

Facilities

The level of facility available is another important factor in assessing a disabled patient's suitability for anaesthesia. If surgery is to be delivered in a large hospital, with access to in-patient beds and specialist support, then anaesthesia can be offered to virtually all who require it. On the other hand, small, stand-alone units without hospital support cannot offer care to the severely impaired person without reducing safety. Again, the difficult problem of balancing risks and benefits needs to be considered.

Assessment of patients

Why special assessment?

All patients who are to receive anaesthesia should have an assessment beforehand. The amount of information required, and the complexity of the assessment depends on the fitness of the patient and the nature of the intended procedure.

Patients with impairments are much better managed as "day-cases" or outpatients, as there is much less disruption to both them and their carers[8]. However, they do not necessarily fulfil the criteria which are otherwise applied to day-stay patients[9], and might in some instances be expected to experience an increased incidence of post-operative complications related to their concurrent medical problems, although this is not always necessarily the case[10]. However, awareness of potential medical or management problems is needed before further decisions can be made on suitable care.

Problems may effect the heart, mainly with congenital problems, and risks of cyanosis, embolism, heart failure and endocarditis. The lungs may be compromised, with chronic aspiration with pneumonitis and recurrent chest infections, or restrictive problems due to spinal deformities. Chronic aspiration is usually related to regurgitation, due to gastro-intestinal disorders such as hiatus hernia, poor swallowing, poor stomach emptying, and poor compliance with fasting. Many disabled patients have central nervous system disease, including epilepsy, psychiatric problems requiring medication, deafness and blindness, poor co-ordination, paralysis and spastic paresis. There may be musculo-skeletal abnormalities, including abnormal head and neck anatomy. This can lead to a difficult airway for intubation, large tongue, unstable cervical spine, spinal deformities and contractures. Finally, patients often possess poor veins, and may have abnormal connective tissue and muscle.

Common medical management problems include:

- congenital heart problems – cyanosis, embolism, heart failure, endocarditis
- Chronic aspiration – pneumonitis, recurrent chest infections, asthma
- Physical deformities – paralysis, spastic spasticity, musculo-skeletal abnormalities
- Reflux – hiatus hernia, muscle incoordination
- Central nervous system disease – epilepsy, psychiatric illness

Communication is often difficult, with the patient unable to communicate important medical information which is unknown to carers e.g. pain, feeling unwell, or feeling nauseated.

General management problems include:

- Communication – sensory and intellectual impairment
- Poor compliance with fasting – challenge for carers
- Poor venous access – altered local anatomy
- issues over consent – for impaired adults

What do we assess?

It is not easy to make a detailed assessment of patients with disabilities, and it is likely to be costly and time consuming. It is very important to have decided on the level of care you can safely deliver with the available resources before assessing the patient. Your criteria will then dictate which patients you must filter out as unsuitable.

In the unit in which I work, we have a very well equipped day-stay unit, with experienced staff. We do not have access to in-patient beds, except in an emergency. So, what are we looking for? The main question is, are they fit enough for an out-patient anaesthetic in our unit? To answer this question, we must ask "what is fit ?"

The American Society of Anesthesiologists (ASA) has a grading system used to decide fitness for surgery (Chapter 6). It is unfortunately not much use in these circumstances. For day-case anaesthesia, the "ASA" grading of patients deems that they should be completely fit, or have only a minor, non-disabling illness. Many of these disabled patients are ASA III, and therefore are not regarded as "suitable" day-cases.

A more useful assessment is the likelihood of peri-operative complications, considering the patient's state of health.

Some conditions may carry a high risk of morbidity/ mortality, although this has not really been quantified in this group of patients.

The problems which cause us the most concern are:
- Potential airway obstruction, from bleeding or oedema
- Respiratory inadequacy, such as severe kyphoscoliosis
- CNS problems, such as poorly controlled epilepsy
- Cyanotic heart disease

Information is also required about medication, so that appropriate pre-operative instructions can be given. For patients with impairments, all medications should usually be continued on the day of surgery, to minimise disruption to therapy.

Who should do it ?

In an ideal world, the anaesthetist responsible should carry out a full consultation with the patient, and obtain a full history and examine all relevant systems. Unfortunately, the anaesthetist has to delegate most or all of these activities to another member of the team. It is important that the person making assessments is experienced, and able to ask appropriate questions and interpret answers correctly.

Where and how should assessments be made?

The first assessment of any patient who is referred for treatment will be by the clinician providing the dental care. It is vital for assessment of suitability to be commenced at this stage, to minimise the wastage of time and effort later. This implies that the dental clinician that decides to plan for care under general anaesthesia should be aware of the selection criteria of their unit.

The system in use in our unit involves the initial use of a simple medical questionnaire, which is completed in the patients notes on referral. If the patient is deemed potentially suitable for general anaesthesia care within our unit, a further Assessment Form is completed (*Appendix 1*). This contains information relating to medical problems, medication, planned care and likely duration of treatment.

The Assessment Form, with the patients case notes, are then reviewed by the consultant responsible for anaesthesia within the unit. Together, anaesthetist and surgeon then decide, using the information provided, whether the patient is suitable for treatment as a day case. If they are, then they are put onto the waiting list for care. Sometimes, further information is required before a decision can be made, for example, details about a patient's cardiac history or the stability of their epilepsy, and it is sought at this stage.

If all is well, the next assessment is carried out just prior to treatment, when the patient arrives in the unit on the day of the procedure. This assessment is similar to that of any patient presenting for anaesthesia, and similar criteria of suitability are applied. We avoid treating patients with active respiratory infections, or who have not fasted as requested, and so their care is postponed.

Outcome of assessment

Within our unit, the system described here works well, and nearly all of our postponements are for acute respiratory infections. As a measure of morbidity, we have had only one unplanned admission following anaesthesia in over three years, and this was for persistent nausea[10].

Team working

Every individual within our team has a vital role in the safe assessment and care of our patients. It is the team that dictates the level of care that can be delivered safely. However, it is important that all members are flexible, and aware of each others responsibilities.

References

1. Nunn J H. Childhood disability. In: *Paediatric Dentistry*. Welbury R R (ed). Oxford University Press, 1997.
2. van Grunsven M F, Koelen M A. Psycho-social aspects of dental care for the handicapped. An investigation into dental care for handicapped children living at home. *Nederlands Tijdschrift voor Tandheelkunde* 1990; **97:** 448–451.
3. Bettelli G, Guilietti MP , Bitelli G, Iseppi D, Caproni G, Saetti A, Sentimenti F, Vernole B. Handicapped patients. General anaesthesia or sedation? *Dental Cadmos* 1990; **58:** 83–86, 89–93.
4. Muller-Herzog R, Brandts A, Lindorf H H. 10 years of out-patient dental surgery using endotracheal anaesthesia. Research report from dental practice. *Deutsche Zahnärtztliche Zeitschrift* 1992; **47:** 40–41.
5. Murray J J. General anaesthesia and children's dental health: present trends and future needs. *Anaes Pain Control Dent* 1993; **2:** 209–216.
6. Maestre C. The use of general anaesthesia for tooth extraction in young handicapped adults in France. *Br Dent J* 1996; **180:** 297–302.
7. Holt R D, Chidiac R H, Rule D C. Dental treatment for children under general anaesthesia in day care facilities at a London dental hospital. *Br*

Dent J 1991; **170:** 262–266.

8. Nunn J H, Davidson G, Gordon P H, Storrs J. A retrospective review of a service to provide comprehensive dental care under general anaesthesia. *Spec Care Dent* 1995; **15:** 97–101.

9. The Royal College of Surgeons of England. *Report of a Working Party on Guidelines for Day Case Surgery.* Commission on the Provision of Surgical Services.

10. Enever G R, Sheehan J, Nunn J H. A comparison of Post-operative morbidity following outpatient dental care under general anaesthesia in paediatric patients with and without disabilities. *Int J Paed Dent* (In Press).

11. Miyazawa H, Namba H, Seiki K, Karasawa H, Imanischi T, Takeuchi T, Hayashi N, Hirose I. Dental treatment under general anaesthesia. *Shoni Shikagaku Zasshi* 1990; **28:** 1117–1124

12. Manley P C, Pahl J M. Dental services for children with mental handicaps: policy changes and parental choices. *Br Dent J* 1989; **167:** 163–167.

13. Nunn J H, Murray J J. Dental health of handicapped children; results of a questionnaire to parents. *Community Dent Health* 1990; **7:** 23–32.

Dental Care under Day-Stay General Anaesthesia

Anaesthetist approved (signature)   Special Requirements

Likely case length

PATIENT'S NAME: HOSPITAL NO:

DOB: DATE:

HOME ADDRESS:

POST CODE:

TELEPHONE NUMBER:
Alternative telephone number (*for contact in case not available on home number during 9–5*)

USUAL ADDRESS: (*if different from above*)

NAME AND ADDRESS OF GMP:

NAME AND ADDRESS OF GDP:

REFERRING DENTIST (DH):

TRANSPORT TO BE USED FOR DAY STAY VISIT:
Private car   *Taxi*   *Ambulance*

MAJOR PRESENTING COMPLAINT:

IF SYNDROME, LIST FEATURES PRESENT IN THIS PATIENT:

IF SIGNIFICANT, RELEVANT MEDICAL CONDITION
PLEASE DETAIL:

EFFECT ON PATIENT:

TREATMENT/INVESTIGATIONS CARRIED OUT (*if possible, attach letter from Consultant with diagnosis, results of investigations etc*)

CURRENT MEDICATION:

PREVIOUS GA:

PATIENT'S WEIGHT:

ANY RELEVANT FAMILY/SOCIAL HISTORY:

OUTLINE OF PROPOSED DENTAL TREATMENT:

PLEASE DETAIL SPECIAL REQUIREMENTS (*eg x-rays in Theatre, ABC, nasal tube vital, etc*).

Chapter 8

Impairments – Diagnosis and Management

Kari Storhaug

Almost any impairment or disability may be of importance for the choice of preventive regimes, planning and implementation of dental treatment and assessment of outcome. A number of chronic medical conditions and their implications for oral health and treatment procedures will be described in this chapter.

Asthma

Asthma is a common condition which affects around 2% of people in Europe and North-America. In children asthma is commonly caused by allergy. It is important to know what substances the patient reacts to in order to avoid exposure during treatment.

Common allergens in the dental clinic are latex (gloves), nickel in filling materials or steel crowns and substances in certain fluoride varnishes (colophonium). If the patient is allergic to wound plasters such varnishes should be avoided.

Many drugs used for the treatment of asthma may have a negative effect on oral health, either due to their sugar content (syrup, inhalation powders), or because of an effect on salivary secretion or composition. Asthmatic patients using inhaled steroids may be predisposed to oral candidal infections.

If surgical treatment is needed an adjustment of steroid medication prior to treatment may be required.

There is evidence now of a link between asthma and dental erosion (*Figure 1*). Patients who have asthma are more likely to wheeze and cough and thus gastric reflux may be encouraged. Conversely, patients with gastric reflux may inhale stomach contents and these irritate the airway, predisposing to 'asthma' type symptoms. Either way, patients may present with signs of erosion as a consequence of the reflux.

General anaesthesia should be avoided and oral care accomplished under nitrous oxide sedation should an adjunct to local anaesthesia be necessary.

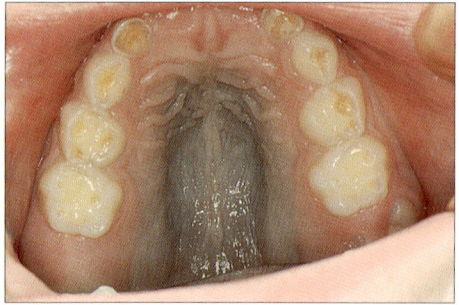

Figure I

Enamel erosion of maxillary primary molar teeth in a child with asthma. Palatal bruising from inhaler trauma.

Figure 2

Finger clubbing in a man with cystic fibrosis.

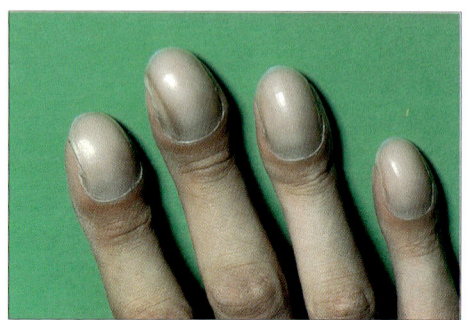

Cystic fibrosis

This is a genetically determined condition which affects exocrine glands. The condition is inherited as an autosomal recessive disease with an incidence of 1:2,500 among caucasians. This is the commonest inherited disease in this ethnic group. Median survival for children with CF used to be one year of age in the 1940s but is now 30 years. Underdiagnosis is common; in one American series 1 in 10 patients were not diagnosed until adult life and in a European series the figure was 1 in 6.

Main presenting signs and symptoms, which may not be present in all are:

Children	Adolescents/Adults
Bowel obstruction	As for children plus:
Prolonged neo-natal jaundice	asthma
Haemorrhagic disease of the newborn	Bronchiectasis
Recurrent chest infection/wheeze	Nasal polyps
Failure to thrive if pancreatic insufficient	Severe sinusitis
Chronic diarrhoea	Liver disease
Rectal prolapse	Finger clubbing (*Figure 2*)
Electrolyte disorders	
Severe gastro-oesophageal reflux	

There is, as a consequence, progressive lung damage such that patients may in time require a heart-lung transplant. One-year survival is around 80% and three-year survival approximately 50% but with poorer results for children. Dentally, older patients still bear the hallmarks of tetracycline therapy with stained teeth.

Dental care is a priority for three reasons:
- a diet high in non-milk extrinsic sugars to maintain calories since fat is not easily metabolised because of pancreatic insufficiency
- saliva production is diminished as is its role in lubrication and buffering
- sweetened medicines may predispose to dental caries and erosion

Bleeding disorders

A defect in any of the factors affecting blood coagulation may affect haemostasis. The most common conditions are haemophilia A (factor VIII), B (factor IX), haemophilia C (factor XI) and von Willebrand disease. Idiopathic thrombocytopenic purpura is another cause of haemorrhage. Typically, a purple rash occurs over mucosal surfaces and the rest of the body following a viral illness. Remission usually follows although recurrences may occur.

Bleeding disorders are rare, often congenital conditions, haemophilia occurring in males as a sex-linked recessive trait. Oral health care should be optimal from an early age to avoid the need for tooth extractions.

Local anaesthesia should be used only in consultation with the patient's physician. If necessary, intraligamentary injections are recommended. If extractions are needed hospitalisation or close co-operation with the patient's haematologist is necessary for administration of factor replacement, DDAVP and Tranexamic acid. Fifteen per cent of patients develop antibodies to factor VIII after repeated replacement so that avoidance of the need for this form of cover by rigorous dental prevention is desirable.

Specific dental considerations are:
- rubber dam isolation to protect tissues
- care with high-volume aspirators on the floor of the mouth – protect by use of gauze over the orifice
- supra-gingival crown and orthodontic band margins
- avoidance of electrocautery because of delayed bleeding after clot lysis
- Tranexamic acid mouthwashes to control gingival oozing to aid oral hygiene
- pulpotomies in preference to extractions – control bleeding with 1:1000 adrenaline

- avoid aspirin and NSAIDs for pain relief as such drugs aggravate the bleeding tendency.

Cardiovascular disorders

Most cardiovascular disorders develop in adult life, but around 1% of children have a congenital heart defect.

Many children with congenital heart disease may need endocarditis prophylaxis before dental procedures which may cause bleeding. Therefore preventing oral diseases in children with heart disease should have high priority. Infective endocarditis accounts for just over 200 deaths per year in England and Wales with a 25% mortality from infective endocarditis, an incidence that has not changed in a decade. For adults, invasive dental procedures should be avoided in the first 6 months after heart surgery or myocardial infarction.

Patients with pace-makers or defibrillators do not require endocarditis prophylaxis.

Patients who do require prophylaxis are:

- Patients with a history of rheumatic fever – usually in the 50+ age group
- congenital cardiac disorders
- cardiac murmurs – with regurgitation
- coronary artery bypass (CABG)
- cardiac valve replacement

When in doubt, consultation with the patient's heart specialist is strongly recommended.

Current recommendations for endocarditis prevention

Mouth rinse with chlorhexidine prior to treatment.
Children: 50 mg amoxicillin per kg body weight
Adults: 3 g amoxicillin.

In both cases the drug should be given as a single dose 1 hour prior to treatment. In cases of allergy to penicillin, clindamycin can be used.

For patients who are allergic to these drugs or who are being treated under general anaesthesia, the guidelines issued by a country's antimicrobial prophylaxis group should be consulted.

Patients who have undergone cardiac and cardiac/lung transplants are a priority group for oral and dental care.

Transplantation is usually the only treatment for patients who have:

- severe ischaemic disease in a young person (familial hyperlipidaemia)

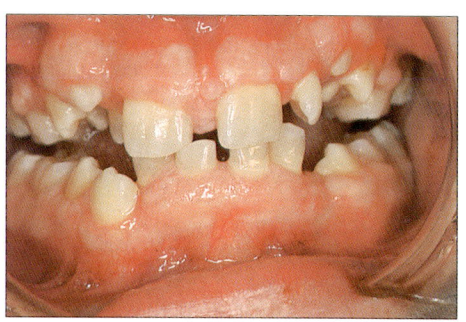

Figure 3
Post-transplant drug-induced gingival enlargement

- cardiomyopathy
- cardiac valve disease
- severe congenital malformation

Pre-transplant all necessary dental work should be undertaken to eliminate any likely sources of infection. However, the patient may well be in an ASA IV state and unable to cope with extensive care, Sedation and especially general anaesthesia will be contraindicated. Teeth of poor prognosis, those with periapical areas and inadequate periodontal support should be removed. Warfarin therapy will preclude extraction unless the INR can be reduced to between 2–4.5. Sockets should be packed and sutured.

Post-transplant, patients will be taking a variety of drugs to manage both the cardiac condition and any underlying condition that may have precipitated the need for the transplant, for example, cystic fibrosis.

Drug types in use with patients who have had heart/lung transplants:
- immunosuppressants, nowadays FK506 which produces less renal toxicity
- corticosteroids
- diuretics
- coronary and peripheral vasodilators
- ACE inhibitors

Post-transplant dental care needs to pay particular attention to the increased likelihood of infection, especially fungal, as a consequence of immunosupression. Patients taking some immunosuppressants and calcium-channel blockers may experience gingival overgrowth (*Figure 3*). In the growing child the overgrowth may be so severe as to impede the eruption of teeth and is unsightly as well as posing problems for cleaning.

Patients who are immunosupressed may develop lymphomas and Kaposi's sarcoma and particularly carcinomas as a consequence of cyclosporin therapy.

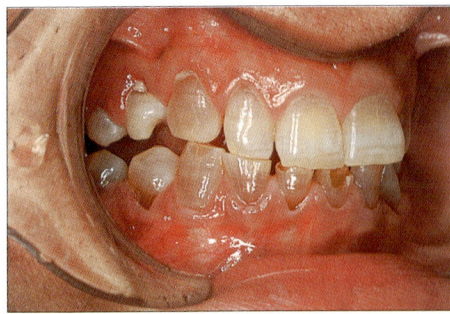

Figure 4

Varying severity of tooth discolouration in OI with dentine aberrations.

Connective tissue disorders

Conditions affecting connective tissue (collagen) have many common features which are of importance for oral health and care.

Specific defects in type I collagen synthesis have been found in many cases. Joint laxity and cardiovascular manifestations as well as craniofacial and dental aberrations are common findings in such conditions, most of which are heritable with varying modes of inheritance, but the frequency of sporadic cases is rather high.

Osteogenesis imperfecta (OI)

This condition, sometimes referred to as brittle bone disease, is a group of disorders with varying severity, causing some of the following: bone fractures, growth retardation and deformity, easy bruising, blue sclerae and loss of hearing. Frequency of OI is reported to be around 1:10,000.

Dentine aberrations resembling dentinogenesis imperfecta or opalescent dentine dysplasia are found in almost 50% of patients (*Figure 4*). Treatment may be complicated by malocclusion (relative mandibular overjet), TMJ-problems and cardiovascular disease.

In the most severe cases steel crowns on primary molars and gold crowns in the permanent dentition may be required to avoid excessive occlusal wear. Extraction of teeth is to be avoided because of the danger of jaw fracture and persistent capillary bleeding. A good preventive regime from early childhood is essential for persons with OI.

Marfan syndrome

Skeletal, cardiovascular and ocular problems are common findings in Marfan syndrome. Patients are usually very tall and slim with long, spider-like fingers and toes. Lens dislocation occurs in around 80% of cases.

Common cardiovascular defects are aortic and pulmonary dilatation and mitral valve prolapse so that the patient requires endocarditis prophylaxis.

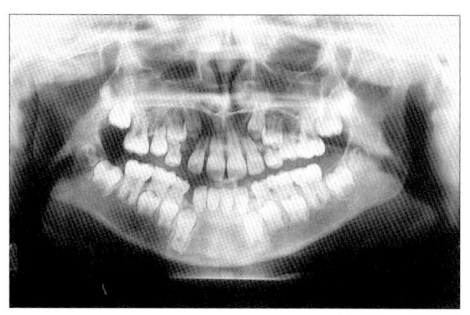

Figure 5
Short roots on lower incisors in EDS

TMJ dysfunction with pain or subluxation may occur during dental treatment. A high and long palatal vault, long slender teeth and malocclusion have been reported.

Ehlers-Danlos syndrome

In this condition extreme hyper-mobility of joints and hyper-extensible skin with slow wound healing and ugly scars are characteristic. Mitral valve prolapse and rupture of large arteries are the most severe cardiovascular complications leading again to the need for antibiotic prophylaxis for invasive dental care. Extraction of teeth may result in prolonged bleeding because of the fragility of blood vessels.

Intraorally, fragile mucous membranes and gingival bleeding after minor trauma (flossing or tooth-brush) are common findings. Prolonged bleeding after tooth extraction may occur. Dental abnormalities include root-deformities (*Figure 5*), and early pulp obliteration/pulp stone formation is common. Effect of local anesthesia may be poor, and intra-ligamental injections are recommended to avoid perforation of vessels.

Ectodermal disorders

Conditions affecting ectodermal tissues like skin, hair, nails and exocrine glands are of particular importance to dentists because teeth (enamel) and salivary glands are of ectodermal origin (*Figure 7*).

Ectodermal dysplasias (ED)

This condition comprise more than 150 different rare, congenital types. Common to all is that at least two ectodermal tissues are affected. There may be hypodontia, oligodontia (more than 6 permanent teeth missing, excluding third molars), and even anodontia (*Figure 6*). Teeth that are present are often small, incisors may have a conical shape, and the enamel layer may be thin. In cases of oligodontia and/or the presence of several conical teeth, possible abberrations in other ectodermal tissues should be assessed and family history taken.

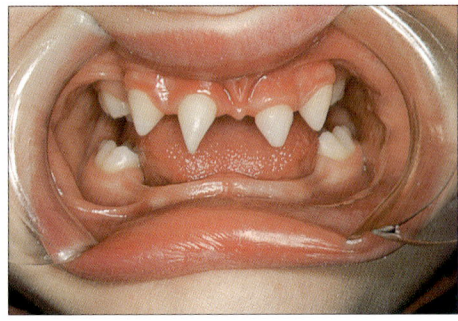

Figure 6
Conical incisors and oligodontia in ED

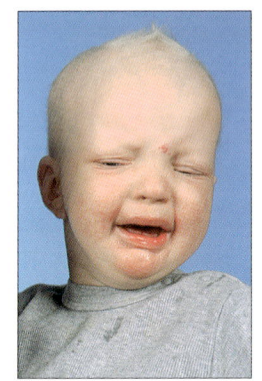

Figure 7
X-linked
anhidrotic ED

The most serious and well-described conditions are the x-linked anhidrotic ectodermal dysplasia (*Figure 7*) and incontinentia pigmenti.

In the x-linked form mothers are carriers, possibly with mild symptoms, while their sons may be severely affected. The lack of sweat glands have serious consequences since fever may result in overheating and death.

Incontinentia pigmenti only affects girls (male foetuses are probably aborted). In additon to missing and conical teeth, skin defects (hyperpigmentation/bullae and hyperkeratosis along lines of Blaschko) are common.

Dentists can contribute to making an early diagnosis in the ectodermal dysplasias.

It is important for children's speech development, chewing ability and self esteem that prosthetic replacement of missing or conical teeth by crowns, dentures and implants are considered at an early age (3–5 years in the most severe cases).

Reduced salivary secretion is common in ectodermal dysplasias. Therefore good preventive regimes should be established early and if indicated, saliva substitutes prescribed.

Epidermolysis bullosa (EB)

This condition affects skin and mucous membranes as well as teeth (enamel). There are several types of EB with varying severity. All are congenital.

In EB simplex, bullae are formed on hands, feet and other skin areas exposed to friction or pressure, like elbows and knees. There is usually no scarring, lesions in the oral mucosa are rare and dental enamel is normal.

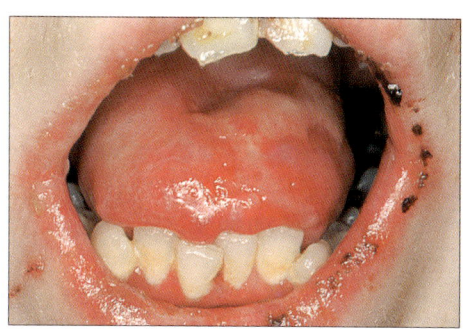

Figure 8
Affected mucous membranes and enamel defects in dystrophic EB

In dystrophic (*Figure 8*) and junctional types of EB, mucous membranes are often affected and scarring may lead to reduced tongue mobility and mouth opening. Dental enamel may be hypomineralised or hypoplastic, and oral hygiene may be difficult to perform due to constant blistering and reduced mouth opening. For some adult patients scarring and contractures can render the hands useless as a means of holding a toothbrush and help from others will be required with this task.

Diluted chlorhexidine/fluoride rinse applied with a soft brush, Q-tips or "Water-Pik" may help maintaining good oral hygiene. Silicone oil applied sparingly will form a thin, protective film over the mucous membranes and protect them from minor trauma during food ingestion. When dental enamel is severely affected, crowning of all permanent teeth may be necessary.

Tuberous sclerosis (TS)

This is a condition which presents as depigmented skin, café-au-lait spots and skin fibromas. Fibromas often form a butterfly pattern over the nose and cheeks. Fibromas may occur in the oral mucosa and in all other organs including the brain, resulting in treatment-resistant epilepsy and mental retardation in some cases.

Characteristic hypoplastic lesions of enamel (enamel pits) are very common in tuberous sclerosis, and detection of pits and intraoral fibromas may be of importance for diagnosis.

Learning disorders

Problems of learning and understanding a complex world may be due to congenital chromosomal aberrations, metabolic conditions, intrauterine infections, trauma or prematurity.

Irrespective of cause, an intellectually impaired individual may have defects, diseases and developmental defects of teeth and jaws which are of importance for oral health care.

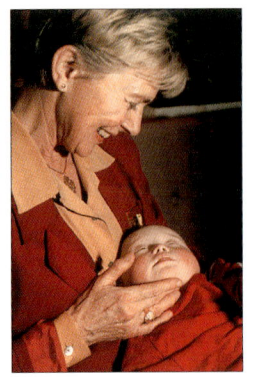

Figure 9

Early stimulation in Down Syndrome

The most common chromosomal anomaly leading to intellectual impairment is trisomy 21, or Down syndrome.

In Down syndrome there may be immunodeficiency, cardiac disease and hypothyroidism. Recurrent respiratory infections are common, and leukaemia is around 10 times more frequent in people with Down syndrome compared to healthy individuals. Early dementia (Alzheimer) is seen in around 50% of individuals with Down syndrome after the age of 40.

Oral/dental characteristics

Babies are often poor suckers due to hypotonia, so breast feeding may be difficult but should be strongly encouraged because of the associated immunodeficiency, the importance for mother/child bonding, for optimal development of the jaws and tongue positioning. Early stimulation of facial and oral muscles may help (*Figure 9*).

Children with Down syndrome who have not been breast-fed will often become habitual mouth breathers with tongue protrusion. Removal of adenoids to facilitate nose breathing and a small palatal plate with a depression near the rear part of the hard palate to create suction to the dorsum of the tongue may be of help before 1 year of age (see chapter 11).

Many dental aberrations related to Down syndrome have been reported. Delayed tooth eruption, conical incisors and small teeth with short roots are often seen, and tooth agenesis is common (*Figure 10*). Early loss of teeth caused by periodontal disease has been reported, but this can be prevented by early intervention, a good oral hygiene regime and frequent follow-up (3–4 times a year) by the dental team.

Relative mandibular prognathism due to a small maxilla is another characteristic trait as is atlanto-axial instability which is of significance for the anaesthetised patient when care in handling is especially important.

Oral/dental anomalies in Down syndrome;

- Relative mid-face hypoplasia
- Tongue protrusion/open mouth posture
- High vaulted palate
- Large, fissured tongue
- Hypodontia
- Hypoplasia
- Microdontia
- Periodontal disease

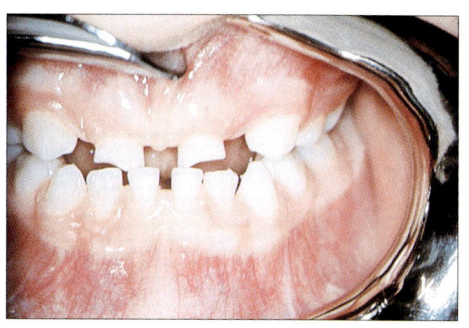

Figure 10
Tooth agenesis and small teeth in Down Syndrome

Most individuals with intellectual impairment can be spared dental disease, loss of teeth and treatment under general anaesthesia if early contact (before the age of 3 years) and regular visits are established.

Fragile-X syndrome

Next to Down syndrome this is the commonest reason for intellectual impairment in males. Relatively under-diagnosed it is of dental significance since a significant proportion will have mitral valve prolapse and will thus require antibiotic prophyaxis for any dental care that breaches the gingival margin.

Neurological disorders

Cerebral palsy (CP) is caused by early brain damage, usually before birth. It is a common cause of physical disability in children, and in around 1/3 of cases there is also a learning disability. A much higher proportion (60-70%) have speech difficulties which may be misinterpreted as a learning disability. The dental team should be aware that most persons with CP have normal intelligence, even if speech is impaired.

Around 1/3 of persons with CP have epilepsy and a considerable proportion have visual problems.

The most common physical result of CP is spasticity with contractures, either hemiplegia (one arm/one leg), quadriplegia (all limbs) or paraplegia (both arms or legs). Athetosis or ataxia are also seen in CP.

Associated conditions are:

- Epilepsy
- Intellectual impairment
- Sensory disorders
- Emotional problems
- Speech and communication disorders
- Altered swallowing reflex

75

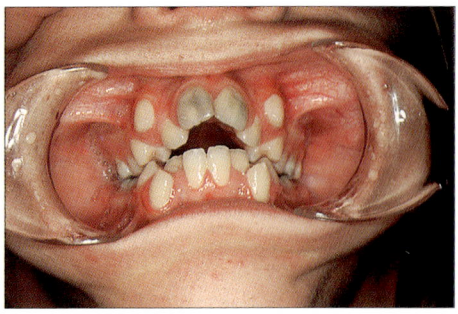

Figure 11
Severe malocclusion on CP

Anxiety in the treatment situation may aggravate spasms. A pleasant, relaxed athmosphere and a correct sitting position with head (not neck!), arm and foot support will prevent increased spasms. Nitrous oxide or benzodiazepine sedation may be useful in some cases.

Dental trauma, malocclusion and drooling are quite common oral health problems in CP (*Figure 11*). Drooling and malocclusion may be reduced by oral stimulation and training from an early age. Daily stimulation for a period of 6–12 months, sometimes palatal plates as well as medication to reduce drooling, should be tried before salivary gland surgery is considered.

Enamel hypomineralisation and hypoplasias occur frequently with CP. Therefore early contact and regular follow-up should be the rule. A battery-operated toothbrush and other technical aids should be tried to facilitate oral hygiene at home.

Dental findings in CP:

- Tongue thrust and mouth breathing
- Malocclusion – class II with anterior open bite
- Drooling/decreased parotid flow rate
- Bruxism
- Increased prevalence of dental caries
- Drug-induced gingival overgrowth
- Enamel hypoplasia
- Dental trauma

Epilepsy

This is a sign, rather than a disease entity in its own right, of underlying organic brain damage that produces abnormal electrical activity in the brain. The results are various: altered levels of consciousness, psychic sensory symptoms, alterations in or absent muscle control. Epilepsy occurs in around 1% of all people, but is more common in persons with learning disabilities and CP. Any form of brain damage

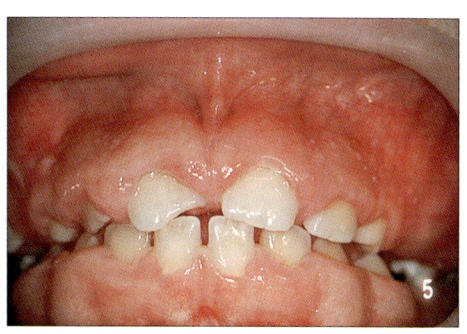

Figure 12

Gingival hyperplasia and tooth trauma in epilepsy

may cause epilepsy in the form of seizures with loss of consciousness (grand mal) or absences (petit mal) which are seen in children.

Major presenting forms of epilepsy:

- Petit mal
- Grand mal
- Staus epilepticus

In most cases epilepsy can be controlled by medication, and there are no problems for the dental practitioner. It is important to know the form and frequency of seizures and whether any outside cause may trigger a seizure (anxiety, sharp flashing light etc.).

Dental management concerns:

- Identification of seizure type and characteristics
- Duration of signs
- Trigger factors
- Presence of an aura
- Patient's management strategy
- Post-seizure events

Trauma during seizures may damage teeth and jaws, and if injuries to the face occur frequently, restoration techniques and materials should be selected with care.

It is well known that some antiepileptic drugs cause gingival hyperplasia while others may affect salivary secretion. Good oral hygiene will reduce the side effects of medication.

Dental problems associated with epilepsy (Figure 12):

- dental trauma
- drug-induced gingival hyperplasia
- increased bleeding tendency from some drugs
- dilantin-induced dysplasia of primary and permanent teeth
- Soft tissue lesions, ulceration, and xerostomia consequent on drug therapy

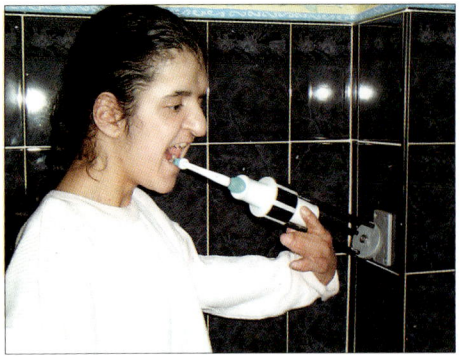

Figure 13

A device to aid the use of a battery-operated tooth brush in an adult with Apert's syndrome and limited manual dexterity

- Poor communication abilities, lack of coordination, learning and emotional disturbances as a result of drug therapy
- malocclusion

Progressive neurological disorders

Multiple sclerosis, Parkinson's disease and progressive neuromuscular conditions are common degenerative disorders in adults.

In all such conditions the ability to carry out daily oral hygiene may be hampered, and electric toothbrushes, other technical aids (*Figure 13*), chemical plaque control (chlorhexidine) and more frequent visits to the dental clinic may be necessary. In late stages of such diseases regular home-visits by a dental hygienist/dental nurse may be useful to avoid pain and deterioration of oral health.

Multiple sclerosis (MS)

This is the most common neurological disease affecting young adults. The condition is more prevalent in Northern Europe and North America.

The aetiology is unknown but may be viral in origin associated with immunologically mediated effects resulting in demyelination and eventually paralysis.

The clinical features are:
- initially visual disturbances and/or limb weakness/paralysis
- nystagmus, ataxia, jerky speech, tremors, loss of muscle co-ordination
- Eventually paralysis with loss of sphincter control and urinary incontinence

Of dental significance is that these patients will intermittently take courses of corticosteroids and/or ACTH. Other drugs used to control bladder dysfunction may result in a dry mouth

Patients presenting with multiple sclerosis may report abnormal perioral sensation – hypersensitivity or anaesthesia. Young patients presenting with signs and symptoms of trigeminal neuralgia particularly bilateral, should be investigated for MS.

Patients, as a consequence of these altered sensations, may have difficulty in localising pain and thus the clinician should be absolutely clear as to the origins of the discomfort before carrying out restorations, extractions or endodontic therapy. As function deteriorates, carers will need to be involved in helping with the oral hygiene routine.

Parkinson's disease (PD)

This is a common disorder, increasing with age, with clinical effects due to the deficiency of the neurotransmitter, dopamine. Males and females are equally affected.

Parkinsonism may also be caused by:
- head injury
- CVA
- dopamine-receptor blocker drugs
- encephalitis
- environmental toxins

The clinical characteristics of the disease are:
- Tremor
- Rigidity
- Abnormal posture leading to stooping
- slowness of movement/lack of spontaneous movement
- shuffling gait
- restlessness
- drooling

The autonomic dysfunction may lead to problems with hypotension, respiratory control and hypersalivation. Anticholinergic drugs used in treatment can cause xerostomia and disorientation as well as interacting with narcotics and antihistamines. Dopaminergic drugs can cause xerostomia, sialorrhoea, nausea, dysphagia and hallucinations and will interact with benzodiazepines and epinephrine.

Dental care appointments should be kept as brief as possible since stress increases tremor. Dental team members should be careful in altering the position of the dental chair too rapidly to avoid orthostatic hypotension.

The mask-like, impassive face of many sufferers belies the ability to communicate normally and dental staff need to be aware of this. The involuntary movements of facial musculature (dyskinesia) place the patient at risk if rotary instruments are used. A mouth prop may help to control some involuntary movements.

Restorations should be kept simple – compatible with the patient's ability at home oral care and new dentures should be avoided. Rather, a denture copy technique should be used if replacement prostheses are required.

Good suction is essential, especially under rubber-dam, to prevent saliva accumulating.

Rheumatic disorders

A large number of adults in Europe and North-America suffer from degenerative musculoskeletal diseases, the most common being osteoarthritis and rheumatoid arthritis (RA).

Degenerative destruction of joints without inflammation is called osteoarthritis, whilst RA is an autoimmune disorder causing inflammation and degeneration of joints. RA also occurs in children, and in the most severe forms may cause growth retardation and deformity.

Many patients with rheumatic disorders have problems carrying out adequate oral hygiene due to hand, wrist, elbow or shoulder involvement, and the oral health care professions should help patients to find ways to overcome problems by means of technical aids, modified toothbrushes and/or chemical plaque control. Some patients with RA use braces for their wrists and fingers and self-care oral hygiene appliances can be adapted to these (see chapter 4).

Good oral hygiene is of importance in RA because around 50% of patients have reduced salivary secretion. Saliva substitutes are not popular among patients, but fluoride tablets or chewing gum may be of help for some. Sjogren's syndrome is more prevalent in patients with RA with all the sequelae of a dry mouth. Patients may need saliva stimulants (where there is residual gland function) or saliva substitutes. There are excellent saliva substitutes available that contain fluoride as well. Care must be used with mouth swabs since many contain agents that will cause dental caries and erosion.

Other dental considerations are:

- Anaemia
- Impaired healing/infection secondary to anti-inflammatory and steroid drugs
- Bleeding secondary to medications
- Cervical spine damage and comfort of dental chairs

In rheumatoid arthritis the temporo-mandibular joint(s) may be affected with pain, reduced joint mobility and occlusion changes as a result (*Figure 14*). This can be dramatic, especially in children where mandibular growth may be hampered. Conservative measures such as

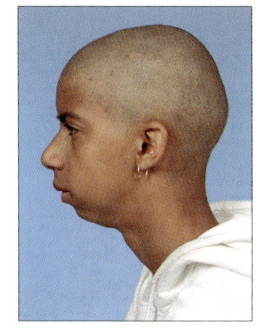

Figure 14

Reduced mandibular growth in JRA

heat, exercises, anti-inflammatory drugs and analgesics may be helpful. In some cases surgical correction can be performed in young adults.

Many children with RA are treated with high doses of steroids and/or cytotoxic drugs. Obliteration of pulp chambers may be seen as a result of such treatment.

Some patients with rheumatic disorders develop more dental disease because of a dry mouth and difficulties with oral hygiene. In such cases an individualised follow-up programme should be offered.

References

1. Scully C, Cawson R A (Eds). *Medical Problems in Dentistry*.
2. Rose L F, Kaye R (Eds). *Internal Medicine for Dentistry*. 2nd edition. The C V Mosby Company, 1990.
3. Jaffe A, Bush A. Cystic fibrosis: a management update. *Prescribers' J* 1999; **39:** 91–96.
4. Thompson A J. Drug therapy in multiple sclerosis. *Prescribers' J* 1999; **39:** 80.
5. Stephen L J, Brodie M J. New drug treatments for epilepsy. *Prescribers' J* 1998; **38:** 98–106.

Chapter 9

Behaviour Management – Children and Adolescents

Gunilla Klingberg

Introduction

Oral care for children and adolescents should aim at prevention and treatment of oral diseases as the basis for good oral health throughout life. This is of special importance when treating young individuals with disabilities due to physical/psychological impairment or chronic disease. Therefore, efforts should be made to ensure that children and adolescents with special needs have the same opportunities as others to develop and maintain good oral health. This includes two issues: first to keep the oral environment healthy, and second to keep the patient capable of, and willing to, utilise the dental service.

All children and adolescents, including children with impairments, show tremendous variation in maturity, personality, temperament and emotions, leading to a corresponding variation in vulnerability and ability to cope with the dental treatment situation[1]. Children and adolescents with mental impairments have different abilities to cope with dental treatment depending on their level of reasoning. Based on Piagetian theories Kylén[2] constructed a model to understand how people with mental developmental impairments reason (*Figure 1*). At level A the person is able to understand the present – here and now; at level B the person's understanding is based on his own experiences; and at level C the person is able to understand and reason about things

Figure 1

Appropriate techniques for dental behaviour management of disabled children and adolescents depending on level of reasoning. Figure illustrates possible techniques when carrying out restorative treatments or extractions. Picture adopted from Alborn & Hallonsten, 1993. The blue line represents development for persons

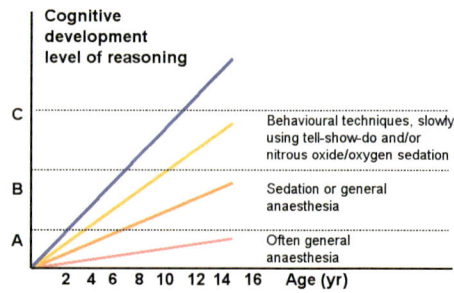

without mental/cognitive disabilities. Coloured lines illustrates development of reasoning for people with disabilities corresponding to the different levels.

that might happen. The majority of people with mental impairments are found at level C. The area above level C represents normal adult reasoning. A person with normal development passes from level A to B at about the age of two, and from level B to C when about seven years old. Level C is passed at the age of 11. This variety in maturity and development in children and adolescents requires the treating dentist to have knowledge regarding many things: different traits in development, medical conditions, different medications etc. In addition to this the dentist should, apart from dental treatment techniques, also know about different behaviour management techniques.

The ability to cope with dental treatment will depend on:
- Level of maturity
- Personality
- Emotions
- Medical conditions
- Developmental stage
- Medication

Creating a safe environment for the patient

Before carrying out any oral treatment the patient must feel safe in the clinical environment.

There are at least three factors, which must be fulfilled for children to feel safe:
- good relationship (rapport) between child, accompanying person and dental team
- no or minimal pain stimuli
- feeling of control.

The communicative competence of the oral team is important when establishing good rapport. All patients have the right to have understandable information about their oral health and required treatments. When meeting disabled children and adolescents the communication must be adapted to the maturity, foremost cognitive abilities, of the person. Adequate communication should also be established with accompanying adults (parents, guardians, nursing staff, and others). This is an absolute prerequisite for compliance. For some patients sign language is needed to ensure communication (*Figure 2*). Small children and children who are intellectually impaired should not be separated from their parents/guardians, since the anxiety this causes may increase their general stress level and decrease the possibility of communication. The patient must never be treated in a patronising way, even if behaviour or attitude are provocative. The child/adolescent must feel a reasonable level of equity in the situation. All treatment must be

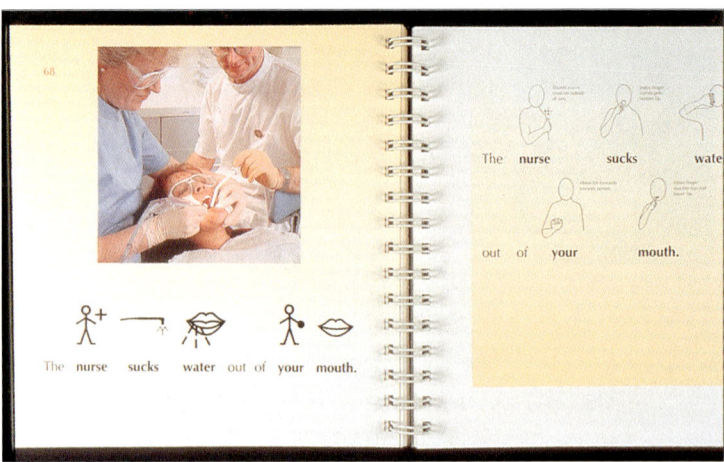

carried out in collaboration with the patient and the patient and/or parent/guardian should give their consent to suggested treatment plans.

In order to feel safe the child must be convinced that the treating oral team will carry out the treatment in a gentle way, avoiding pain and discomfort. Strategies to minimise pain will be dealt with separately, see below.

Feeling of control in the child can be accomplished by information and stepwise introduction to all steps in the treatment, i.e. behaviour shaping. How vulnerable a child or adolescent is when entering the dental clinic depends on personal factors like medical condition, general emotional status, psychological development, temperament, cognitive abilities etc[1]. Further, the social context of the child will influence how the child perceives the situation. Some children and adolescents are more robust and may tolerate a lot, while others are vulnerable and respond negatively even to small stress stimuli. Many children and young people with disabilities and impairments have experienced painful and/or stressful medical as well as oral examinations and treatments leading to lowered tolerance of dental procedures.

Pre-requisites for willingness to undergo treatment:

- rapport
- feeling of safeness
- feeling of being in control
- understanding
- empathetic manner
- good communication with carers
- informed consent

Behaviour shaping

Behaviour shaping of children implies training in how to cope with dental instruments and procedures that they will meet. All children need behaviour shaping in the dental chair, irrespective of their oral vulnerability and potential treatment need. However, the time required for this varies tremendously between different individuals. For some children and adolescents with disabilities, the oral team needs to invest a lot of time in these procedures. An attitude in the oral team characterised by empathy, kindness, encouragement and positive reinforcement serves as a basis for this work.

The most accepted and common type of behaviour shaping in dentistry is based on the concept of exposure therapy. The patient is exposed to potential anxiety provoking instruments and procedures step by step. Each step creates a moderate increase in stress (and fear), and the exposure is maintained until the patient comes to realise that the fear-provoking event is less so. A feeling of ability to cope with the stimuli is thereby created. The different steps in the behaviour-shaping stairway should be adapted to the individual patient and situation[3]. During each exposure the 'tell-show-do' technique (TSD) is used. The child is first told what will happen, then shown, and finally exposed to the procedure. If the child positively accepts the procedure, its impression of coping must be reinforced by making the child aware of its capability (feedback). If the acceptance is negative, the child should be met with empathy and given more training on the previous step.

The attention span varies immensely between different child patients. Children and adolescents with disabilities like DAMP (Deficit in Attention and Motor control and Perception) and ADHD (Attention Deficit, Hyperactivity Disorder) are common encounters in the dental clinic. Prevalence figures up to 8% for DAMP and 4% for ADHD have been reported from Sweden. These children need a calm environment in the dental clinic in order to be able to co-operate. Stimuli like noise or music from a radio, a telephone ringing, somebody entering the room, too many toys or pictures in the room etc. lead to distraction and prevents the child from focusing on the oral treatment and the communication with the oral team. It is, therefore, a good thing to minimise these stimuli. These patients need dental staff that have lots of patience and who are prepared to put a lot of effort into introducing the treatment, often in very small steps and working hard on keeping the child's focus on the treatment.

Body posture

A clinical situation where the child patient is able to relax in the dental chair is if not a prerequisite, at least an ideal basis for good manage-

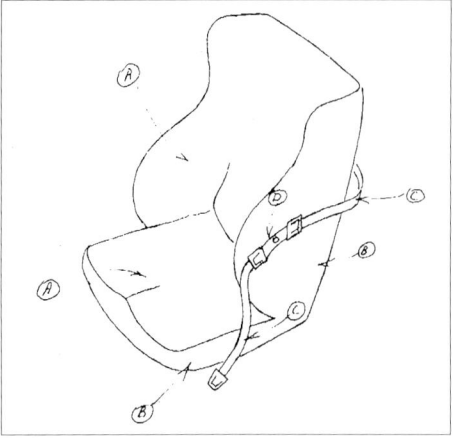

Figure 3

A body support to aid in the treatment of an impaired young person in the dental chair

ment and oral treatment. The dental chairs normally used are not shaped/constructed for short bodies and are, therefore, both uncomfortable for the child patient to lie in, and also create a problem for the treating dental staff to work in good ergonomic positions. To help this, different sizes and forms of cushions can be used to make the dental chair more comfortable and to support the child's body in a better way. Especially for children with spasticities, cushions can help to create a body posture that decreases/eliminates problems that otherwise might interfere with the oral treatment (*Figure 3*)

Pain-free treatment

Several studies have reported that painful dental treatments are one of the most important causes of dental anxiety and behaviour management problems. Further, there are many reports of an under-use of local anaesthesia in children. Unpublished data from Sweden indicate that the use of local anaesthesia is even less frequent when treating disabled and impaired child patients. The International Association for the Study of Pain defines pain as an unpleasant experience, which is caused by the damage of tissue, or by the threat of such damage[4]. Thus, painful sensations do not necessarily depend upon tissue damage. Pain may also be generated by conditioned stimuli such as the sound of the drill or a gentle touch of the needle.

Children's understanding of, and vulnerability to, pain varies considerably depending on cognitive abilities, and the reactions and thoughts concerning painful stimuli vary according to age and maturity[5]. One strong painful dental stimulus could be enough to cause dental fear and anxiety in a child patient or behaviour management problems. However, repeated exposure to oral treatments that are only somewhat discomforting or a little painful, or perceived as such by the child, can also have the same result. Further, discomfort goes hand in hand with pain and is often experienced in novel situations if the child is frightened about what will happen, or feels a lack of control. Children frequently have problems in distinguishing between pain and discomfort. When treating children and adolescents with impairments and disabilities great efforts should be made to minimise both pain and discomfort. It is not acceptable from an ethical point of view that local anaesthesia is withheld especially as this is a documented way to reduce or even abolish pain[6].

It is wise to ensure that the child patient has a number of pain-free appointments without any unpleasant events prior to experiencing treatments where there is even a minor risk of discomfort or pain. Repeated successful and pain-free dental visits can 'vaccinate' the child against dental anxiety. This latent inhibition of dental fear and anxiety may serve as a good motive for providing regular oral care, preferably focusing on the maintenance of good oral health. Unfortunately, some treatments could be perceived as painful, e.g. injection of local anaesthesia in the palate. Prior to any possibly painful events the dentist must, apart from using techniques to reduce pain, inform the child about what can be expected. The dentist should take time to explain to the child what is going to happen and what will be felt during as well as after injection. The injection procedure should then be introduced using tell-show-do method. Avoid over-dramatisation of syringe and needle demonstration. It is also important that both patient and accompanying adults are informed concerning avoidance of self-inflected bite-wounds in tissues that are anaesthetised.

In order to minimise discomfort and pain a topical application of local anaesthesia should be used, e.g. application of a 5% lidocain ointment or 20% benzocaine on the oral mucosa for at least two minutes. The solution of local anaesthesia should be at room temperature. A gentle injection technique where the local anaesthesia is injected slowly using sharp, thin needles (30 G or 27 G) minimises the risk of pain when administering the solution. It has been reported that children experience less discomfort and pain during injection when the dentist takes time to give the injection. It should take at least two minutes, preferably longer time, to administer 1.8 ml of solution. In order to further acclimatise the patient, a slight finger pressure could be applied to the mucosa just prior to injection followed by aspiration and then a gentle injection of just a few drops. These are allowed to have effect before the rest of the solution is slowly injected. Distraction like e.g. counting to ten at slow pace or telling a short story can also be useful. Some dentists report success from a technique of getting the child to breathe through one nostril and then the other as a potent distractor.

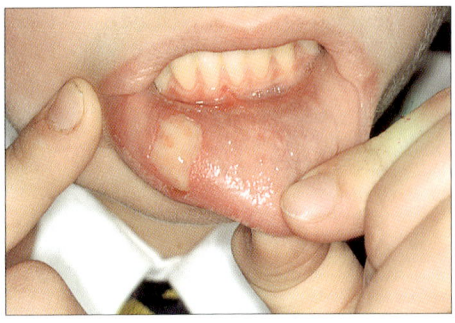

Figure 4

Soft tissue trauma after child bit lip after LA administration

When treating disabled/impaired young patients there are some considerations that have to be made concerning local anaesthesia. For the majority of these patients the strategies are the same as for others. However, in some cases strong negative reaction can be expected after injection, mainly due to the perceived numbness, or there is risk of the patient hurting himself in terms of inflicting bite-wounds (*Figure 4*). This could occur in for example intellectually impaired patients. In these cases a periodontal ligament injection or use of mepivacain could be useful. If this is not an option, the dentist should consider performing treatment under sedation or general anaesthesia. From an ethical point of view it is not acceptable to carry out any treatment that may cause pain, e.g. restorative treatments, without local anaesthesia. Electro-analgesia and intra-osseus injections are new methods still in development. It is very plausible that these techniques may be valuable when treating disabled patients.

Good local anaesthesia technique relies on:

- Equipment out of sight
- Appropriate terminology at the patient's level of understanding
- Adequate surface anaesthesia
- Warm solutions
- Fine gauge needles
- Slow injection technique
- Appropriate distraction

For more complicated treatments like surgery, or if postoperative pain is expected, the patient could receive analgesics as premedication. Analgesics could also be used in situations where the patient has toothache or acute pain due to, for example, traumatic injuries. The most commonly used analgesic for children is paracetamol, which should of course be prescribed in a sugar-free formulation. Other substances that have become available for children in good health are diclofenac and ibuprofen (both from the age of six in Scandinavia). Paracetamol and diclofenac are also reported to be very effective when used together for treatment of postoperative pain in children.

Sedation

The basis for the dental management of impaired/disabled children and adolescents is behavioural techniques. In some cases this is not enough to manage the patient and other techniques have to be used[6-9]. *Figure 1* shows how different techniques can be applied depending on the child's/adolescent's ability to reason.

Conscious sedation implies that the patient is able to independently maintain his airway, independently maintain an open mouth, and respond sensibly to verbal commands. The patient will also retain adequate function of protective reflexes, such as the laryngeal reflex. Conscious sedation in dental child patients can be achieved by a drug's administration orally, rectally, or by inhalation.

Sedation by intravenous administration of, for example, propofol has been reported to be very effective when treating impaired/disabled young patients. As this form of sedation imposes less physical and mental stress on the patient than general anaesthesia this mode of treatment has a special place in the treatment of disabled children and adolescents. Administration of midazolam (orally, rectally or intra-nasal) has been used in adolescents to gain sufficient cooperation to obtain IV access. Dental procedures like oral examination, radiographic examinations, preventive treatments such as fissure sealants, restorative treatment of smaller cavities, can be carried out under intravenous sedation.

The choice of method for sedation should be based on treatment needs, medical status and medication, type of impairment, expected pain, and level of anxiety. When using sedation information to patient and accompanying parent/care taker/guardian concerning effects of sedation, expected reactions, duration etc. is very important. Treatment with sedation must never be carried out unless informed consent is obtained from patient and/or parent.

The main objective for the use of sedation in dentistry for impaired/disabled children and adolescents is to provide light but sufficient sedation in order for the patient to co-operate and be more easily influenced by the behavioural techniques. This is very valuable when introducing intellectually impaired patients in particular to oral treatments and when carrying out preventive dental care. Sedation could also be used in cases where the oral treatment is expected to be particularly stressful. Complicated or lengthy treatments are examples of this. Invasive treatments in very young children or intellectually impaired children that are not able to understand why treatment is carried out is

Table 1. The American Society of Anesthesiologists' (ASA) physical status classification

Classification	Description
Class I	A healthy patient
Class II	A patient with mild systemic disease
Class III	A patient with severe systemic disease that is not incapacitating
Class IV	A patient with incapacitating systemic disease that is a constant threat to life
Class V	A moribund patient not expected to survive for 24 hours with or without operation.

another indication. For some medically impaired patients the stress caused by the treatment and the resultant adrenaline secretion can be a risk factor in cardiac conditions. In some of these cases sedation may be indicated. Further, patients with spasticity and tremor can be helped by use of sedation as can patients with a pronounced gag reflex.

Benzodiazepines are today the drugs of choice when looking at oral administration of tranquillisers. These are also available as rectal preparations. The most commonly used substances in Scandinavian dentistry are diazepam and midazolam. Other substances are oxazepam, lorazepam, nitrazepam, and flunitrazepam. The patients should be assessed according to ASA classification (see *Table 1*). The dentist may take responsibility for treating children and adolescents in Classes I and II, while patients in Classes III and IV should be decided about in consultation with the patients physician. Myasthenia gravis and porphyria are absolute contraindications.

Types of sedation in young, impaired people:

- Oral
- Intra-nasal
- Rectal
- Inhaled
- Intravenous

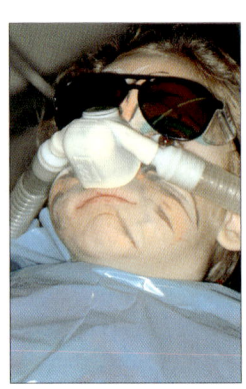

Figure 5

A relaxed child (with face paint – not a skin condition!) undergoing dental care under nitrous oxide sedation

Nitrous oxide/oxygen sedation

Nitrous oxide/oxygen sedation requires that the patient is able to co-operate and breathe through a nasal mask (*Figure 5*). The same considerations concerning ASA classifications as for benzodiazepines should be applied for nitrous oxide/oxygen.

Contraindications to nitrous oxide sedation related to ASA groups I and II:

- partial obstruction of the respiratory airways
- psychosis

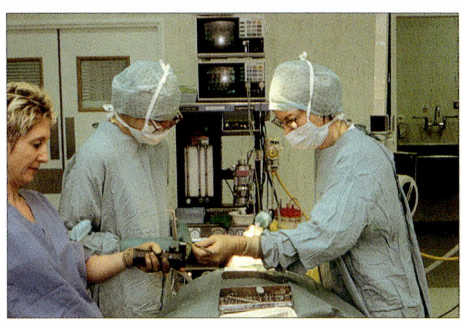

Figure 6

*Dental care under general anaesthesia –
expensive in terms of number of staff
and the sophistication of facilities
required.*

- pregnancy
- recent otological operations/ sinusitis
- porphyria
- malignant hyperthermia in the family

The advantages of nitrous oxide/oxygen sedation are that it is possible to easily adjust the dose and that there is only a short time required for elimination of the gases, i.e. the patient will be fully recovered within a few minutes after administration is terminated. The technique has a wide safety margin and is unlikely to render the patient unconscious unintentionally. Thus, nitrous oxide/oxygen sedation may very well be used in combination with behavioural techniques for many groups of disabled children and adolescents, for example, combined with tell-show-do technique when learning to cope with dental procedures, and for chair-side preventive treatments[9]. Further, nitrous oxide/oxygen sedation reduces spasticities and has, therefore, a special indication for use in these patients.

General anaesthesia

Some patients with physical or intellectual impairments are not able to co-operate during conventional treatment or under sedation. For these patients as well as for patients who for some reason do not tolerate local anaesthesia, treatment under general anaesthesia is indicated. It is important that facilities are available for this form of treatment. Population-based studies from Sweden have reported that 0.2% of the total child population up to the age of nineteen requires dental treatment under general anaesthesia. Children and adolescents that needed this treatment because of disabilities/impairments accounted for 20–34% of the cases treated under general anaesthesia during a period of ten years. The indications for dental treatment under general anaesthesia are wider for children with impairments compared with others. As general anaesthesia exerts great physical and mental stress on the person and is also expensive (*Figure 6*), it is of the utmost importance that the oral care for disabled children and adolescents focuses on prevention. The main objective for oral care of disabled children and adolescents must be good oral health.

Conclusions

- Oral and dental care of children and adolescents with disabilities due to physical/psychological impairment or chronic disease should focus on gaining and maintaining good oral health.
- Always aim at pain-free treatment.
- Invest time in the patient to create a safe environment.
- Behaviour shaping, tell-show-do method, is the basis for most treatments.
- Sedation by use of benzodiazepines or nitrous oxide/oxygen serves as a good complement for treating many patients.
- General anaesthesia should be available to patients who are otherwise not able to cope with oral treatments.

References

1. Klingberg G. Dental fear and behaviour management problems in children. A study of measurement, prevalence, concomitant factors, and clinical effects. Thesis. Faculty of Odontology, Göteborg University, Sweden. *Swed Dent J* 1995; suppl 103.
2. Kylén G. *Begåvning och begåvningshandikapp*. Ala/Handikappinstitutet; 1981.
3. Holst A. Behaviour management problems in child dentistry. Frequency, therapy and prediction. Thesis. Faculty of Odontology, University of Lund, Malmö, Sweden. *Swed Dent J* 1988; suppl 54.
4. International Association for the Study of Pain, Subcommittee on Taxonomy. Pain terms: a list with definitions and notes on usage. *Pain* 1979; **6:** 249–252.
5. Schechter N L, Berde C B, Yaster M (Eds). *Pain in infants, children, and adolescents*. Baltimore: Williams & Wilkins; 1993.
6. Koch G, Modeér T, Poulsen S, Rasmussen P (Eds). *Pedodontics – A Clinical Approach*. Copenhagen: Munksgaard; 1991.
7. Alborn B, Hallonsten A-L. *Handikapptandvård*. Karlshamn: Invest-Odont, LIC Förlag AB; 1993.
8. Welbury R R (Ed). *Paediatric Dentistry*. Oxford: Oxford University Press; 1997.
9. Hallonsten A-L. Nitrous oxide-oxygen sedation in dentistry. Thesis. *Swed Dent J* 1982; suppl 14.

Chapter 10

The Use of Sedation in the Treatment of People with Disability

Graham Manley and Meg Skelly

Introduction

The provision of comprehensive dental care for people with disability involves treatment strategies other than the use of local anaesthesia. It has been suggested[1] that approximately 20% of people with a disability need a general anaesthetic for dental treatment. General anaesthesia is a valuable option in certain cases although there are a number of associated problems. Unless full intubation facilities are available conservative dentistry is difficult, with the consequence that an extraction-only service may be provided. With the use of tracheal intubation the range of treatment options is extended although this may not be comparable with treatment of the conscious patient. For example, multi-visit periodontal treatment, preventive care, some endodontic treatment and certain aspects of advanced conservation, may not be practical under general anaesthetic. Such limitations reduce the availability of treatment options and may result in an overall poorer quality of care. For the person with a disability this may further compound their disadvantage, particularly if there are aesthetic implications such as those due to extraction rather than root treatment of anterior teeth. Society today advocates equal standards of care for all groups[2] and it could be suggested that such problems in the provision of dental care provide a handicap rather than remove one.

In addition to these problems, orofacial pathology may be one of many possibilities that result in painful symptoms and a significant change in behaviour. This may be particularly difficult in patients with limited ability to communicate. Self injury or aggressive physical violence to others may result from frustration due to the individual's inability to indicate the source of pain or failure to cope. General anaesthesia may be considered to be the only way of carrying out an examination to exclude dental caries or other orofacial pathology as the reason for these problems and, subsequently, to provide treatment. If no orofacial pathology is discovered, the use of general anaesthesia, a procedure not without risks, might seem to have been unwarranted. The question also arises as to whether people with challenging behaviour, or a severe learning disability, should be given a general anaesthetic for a routine dental check in the absence of symptoms. However, it should be recognised that in a properly controlled situation, with the appropriately trained, qualified and experienced staff, the risk to patients receiving treatment under general anaesthesia is small[3] unless there are complicating medical conditions[4].

A number of reports[5–7] have encouraged the use of sedation as an alternative to general anaesthesia. Sedation is considered to be safer and more likely to be available in the primary care setting. It offers the opportunity for multiple appointments and a wide range of treatment options. The use of sedation may therefore address many of the problems associated with general anaesthesia.

Disadvantages of GA-only for dental care in people with impairments:

- need for full intubation if restorative care is to be carried out
- treatment options may be limited
- compromised outcomes for patients
- morbidity
- mortality
- cost
- examination may reveal no treatment need

This chapter will consider sedation for people with disability, and the various techniques that have been used in this particular group of patients. An examination of the literature is presented in summary table form (Table1) and a novel technique used for people with particular managment problems is introduced.

Sedation for people with severe learning disability / challenging behaviour – assessment

A review of the literature (Table 1) indicates that a variety of techniques and combinations of drugs have been used in the sedation of people with disability. Initial patient assessment will enable a judgement to be made as to the cognitive ability, behavioural co-operation and physical compliance of the patient as well as their medical and social history. The choice of sedation techniques should be the simplest and safest available that is appropriate for the needs of each individual patient. For people with mild or moderate learning disability oral or inhalation sedation may be suitable. The length and or type of procedure may also influence the decision as to the form of sedation. When intravenous sedation is used the operator may also act as the sedationist[25] unless this is contraindicated on manufacturers advice or licence restrictions[26].

Table 1 Literature review

Authors/reference	Drug(s) and route	Subjects and disability	Outcome
Fukata O et al.[8]	Midazolam 0.2 mg/kg intranasal	Learning disability. 21 cases, age 4–23 years	Successful outcome in 70%
Fukata O et al.[9]	Midazolam 0.2mg/kg cf 0.3mg/kg intranasal	Challenging behaviour	No benefits with higher dose. 0.2mg/kg recommended
Manford M et al.[10]	Relative analgesia	Young handicapped	Successful as an alternative to general anaesthesia
Blain K et al.[11]	Relative analgesia	Children	Successful as an alternative to general anaesthesia
Blain K et al.[12]	Relative analgesia	Children	Successful as an alternative to general anaesthesia
Fanning B et al.[13]	Diazepam 10–20mg orally	Children with disability	Cf: oral diazepam with restraint using papoose board. Oral diazepam favourable
Silver T et al.[14]	Midazolam, orally	Children – Physiologically and neurologically compromised, age 3–18 years, 31 cases	60–75% success depending on dosage
Rosenberg M.[15]	Ketamine, orally	'Extremely combative mentally handicapped female'. Case study	Treatment completed successfully
Haney K et al.[16]	Meperidine + promethazine and N_2O/O_2	Medically/physically/ mentally compromised children	Children taking medications with CNS actions – less successful outcomes
Healy T et al.[17]	Diazepam – intravenous and local anaesthetic	Adults with mild to moderate learning disability	Operating conditions successful in 80%
Malamed S.[18]	Intravenous: Diazepam + midazolam + meperidine + pentazocine. Subgroup also intramuscular midazolam + meperidine	Adults with impairments – total 96. Sub-group 14 uncooperative received additional intramuscular combination	Four patients only could not be treated and were referred for general anaesthesia
Oei-Lim L et al.[19]	Propofol (intravenous)	Adults with impairments	Propofol cf. Relative analgesia. Quality and ease of propofol sedation, good. Propofol acceptable alternative to inhalation sedation.
Oei-Lim L et al.[20]	Propofol – computer controlled infusion system (intravenous)	Adults with impairments (med. age 29 yrs). Total 89 ASAI/II	Total (89) unable to treat with relative analgesia. 78 successfully treated using propofol.
Stephens A et al.[21]	Propofol cf. Midazolam (inravenous). Both by continuous infusion (anaesthetist)	People (18) with impairments – age 5–26 years. Double blind crossover	Main advantage of propofol – rapid recovery.
Van der Bijl P et al.[22]	Midazolam (intravenous)	Case study. Patient with spastic nerve muscle disorder. 29 year old female	Successful treatment. Patient had involuntary movements.
Van der Bijl P et al.[23]	Midazolam bolus + propofol infusion (intravenous)	Case study. Patient with learning disability. 21 year old, ASA IV	Treatment extractions. Patient sedated. No significant cardiovascular/resp. effect.
Van der Bijl et al.[24]	Propofol infusion (intravenous)	Case study. Patient with learning disability. 21 year old. ASA IV	Patient well throughout procedure. No adverse effects.

An operator-sedationist must be assisted by a dental nurse trained in the skills of patient monitoring.

Where the patient is unable to understand the nature and implications of treatment and therefore give legal consent, a relative and or carer should be asked to agree that the patient is not able to provide consent and that the treatment is in the patient's best interest. The process of obtaining consent(or at least an agreement to treat) for people with severe learning disability raises a number of legal and ethical issues. It is therefore essential that in addition to a discussion of the dental treatment to be provided, there is a clear understanding of the specific sedation techniques that are proposed. There is, in such cases, a double requirement for consent.

Requirements for delivery of sedation:

- simplest and safest, appropriate technique
- demands of dental procedure to be used
- trained assistant present
- relatives/carers in agreement with proposed treatment plan
- anaesthetist available if indicated by sedation method chosen

Patients with severe learning disability and/or challenging behaviour present particular problems. Verbal communication is rarely possible and behaviour may be strongly physically resistant and aggressive. For such patients inhalation sedation is not possible and intravenous cannulation may be extremely difficult if not hazardous. It is often this group of patients that present with behavioural change which the carers feel may be related to non- specific orofacial symptoms. The use of a general anaesthetic may appear to be the only option for diagnosis and treatment.

Use of a novel combination sedation technique

In response to this particular problem a novel combination sedation technique has been developed. Midazolam is administered orally or intranasally followed by additional intravenous midazolam. Alternatively propofol is administered by a consultant anaesthetist. These methods have enabled patients who had previously received treatment under general anaesthetic to be successfully treated.

A review of this combined sedation technique carried out on patients with severe learning disability/challenging behaviour who were treated in a primary care setting at a community dental health centre is presented. The review examined clinical practice using sedation over a six year period. Results showed an increase in numbers of patients seen with a variation in the use of intravenous propofol or midazolam (*Figure 1*) The use of a combination of oral or intranasal midazolam

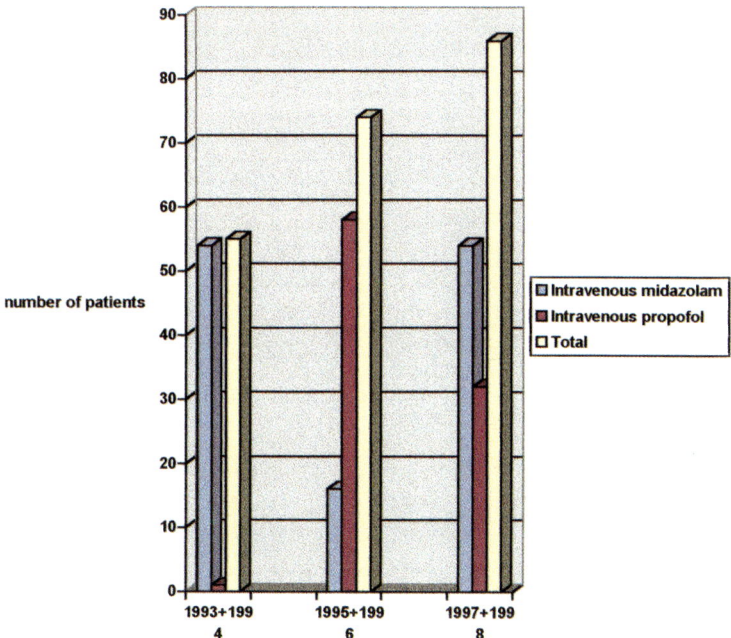

Figure 1

Pattern of sedation by numbers of patients treated over a six year period. Midazolam and propofol were used intravenously

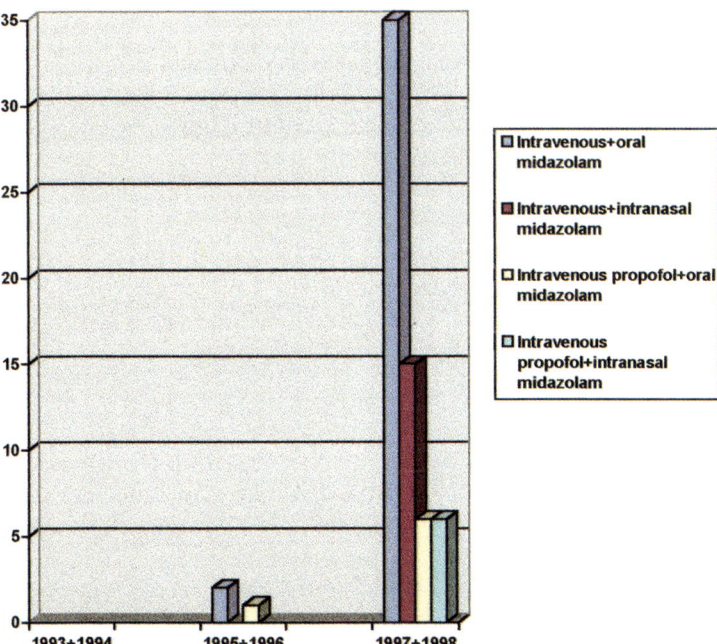

Figure 2

Number of patients treated using a combination of oral or intranasal midazolam with intravenous midazolam or intravenous propofol

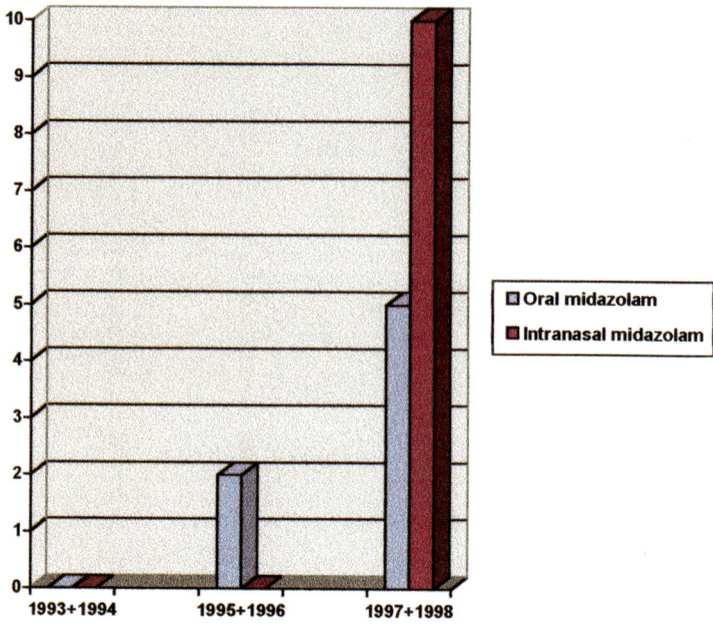

with intravenous midazolam increased markedly (*Figure 2*). Oral or intranasal use without additional intravenous administration (*Figure3*) was also found to be a valuable technique.

The patients treated were all over 16 years of age, 95% being ASA I+II, 5% ASA III. Most patients were taking medication (92%), and of these the majority (83%) were receiving antiepileptics. The mean number of appointments for treatment per person was 1.5 and midazolam was used orally 102 times over the six year period and intranasally on 62 occasions.During this period only four patients could not be treated using these techniques described and required referral for general anaesthesia.

Midazolam or Propofol?

The choice between the use of propofol and midazolam may depend on a number of factors. First, whether any previous record indicates that the patient had responded better to sedation with one or other drug and, second, whether an additional clinician trained in anaesthetics is available to administer propofol. Propofol may be avoided in patients taking anticonvulsant medication in accordance with information included in the manufacturer's data sheet[26] although there is evidence that such use is not contraindicated[27].

Propofol is of particular value for short procedures (less than 10 minutes) but is also satisfactory for longer cases. Midazolam provides excellent anxiolysis accompanied by sedation. In the case of propofol the levels of anxiolysis and sedation do not necessarily coincide. For some difficult cases propofol provides the option of temporarily increasing the depth of sedation if necessary. The distinction between a satisfactory level of consciousness and deep sedation would appear to be achieved more consistently using midazolam. It seems therefore that midazolam offers a greater margin of safety for conscious sedation than propofol. Comparison between the two drugs has been made in previous work[22] and these comments are made from clinical observations rather than objective assessment.

Choice of drug for sedation depends on:
* patient's previous experience with drugs in use
* availability of an anaesthetist if indicated from drug selected
* degree of anxiolysis and sedation required
* length of dental procedure

Oral and intranasal midazolam

Although the administration of midazolam via the oral or intranasal route is licensed for use in parts of Europe, within the United Kingdom there is no such licence in operation. The off-licence use of a drug is accepted as a right of the practising clinician[28], but it is important that a number of procedures are followed[29,30].

Mention should be made about the off-licence use of midazolam on the consent form and all those involved in the treatment process informed accordingly. The suppliers of the drug should be aware of, and in agreement with, the off-licence use of this drug.

As part of the professional's justification to use a drug in this way a considerable body of clinical evidence should be available to support the case that the use of nasal and or oral midazolam is good clinical practice in the situation for which it is being used.

The difficulty with administering intranasal sedation should not be underestimated particularly with this patient group. Ideally the use of a higher concentration of the drug would enable less solution to be used and this has been shown to be effective[8]. Other research has demonstrated the use of a dinosaur toy in improving acceptability to children who are given intranasal midazolam. The toy is connected to a syringe via a number 21 winged infusion set through a Luer-lock[31].

To avoid administering too large a volume of liquid to people with severe learning disability, the 10 mg in 2 ml preparation of midazolam should be used. This can be administered as a fine aerosol through a 2 ml syringe connected via a blunt needle to a spray nozzle (*Figure 4*).

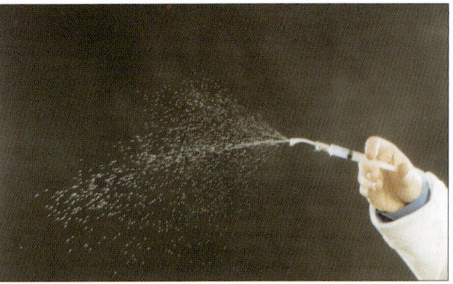

Figure 4

Spray nozzle connected to a 2 ml syringe for the administration of intranasal midazolam

The dose of intranasal midazolam used for adults with severe learning disability/challenging behaviour is 10 mg. If the midazolam is given in fine droplets it is absorbed rapidly and effectively through the nasal mucosa. Other studies[32] have shown an 83% bioavailability via the intranasal route. The average time for effective sedation ranges from four to twelve minutes. The use of midazolam orally also presents problems related mainly to its extremely bitter taste. When administered to patients it is always given in a sweetened drink chosen by the patient. This is usually tea, coffee or fruit juice. The carers accompanying the patient can be also offered refreshment so that the procedure is more of a social rather than a medical/clinical event. The dose of midazolam used orally is generally 20 mg, and the average time for effective onset is twenty minutes.

The availability of the drug has been shown to be about 45%[33] due to the effect of first-pass metabolism in the liver. However, as with the intranasal route, it is usually sufficient to enable the safe and effective placement of a cannula and, in some cases, to complete the treatment required without additional intravenous administration. The benzodiazepine antagonist, flumazenil, may be used electively in some patients. These are cases where it is judged that the patient with challenging behaviour could be more safely managed during the final stages of recovery by the reversal of midazolam rather than with the added problem of residual sedation in a physically difficult-to-manage patient. Where oral or intranasal sedation is used in combination with the intravenous route, the authors have found that the average time from last increment of intravenous drug to discharge is no longer than with intravenous sedation alone (range 35–60 minutes).

Treatment planning and dental care

The types of dental treatment provided using sedation in the review of this novel combined technique included a full range of dental care based on patient needs. These included crowns, endodontic treatment, extensive periodontal therapy, removal of impacted wisdom teeth and other minor oral surgery(apicectomy, surgical exodontia). The priority for treatment planning should be the decisive removal of any possible focus of pain. This does not always necessitate an extraction as might be the case if general anaesthesia is used. Treatment planning depends on the patients response to the sedation provided.

Over a six year period during which these techniques have been used, 25% of patients received repeat courses of treatment. This is higher than one would hope to be the case for patients receiving general anaesthesia. It reflects the value of sedation for regular oral examination of those with challenging behaviour and more regular support for carers by providing periodontal treatment such as scaling.

General anaesthesia or sedation?

The choice between referral for general anaesthetic, and the use of these conscious sedation techniques depends on a variety of factors. Limited availability of intubated general anaesthesia may be a factor. The availability of general anaesthetic and sedation services for people with disability may vary considerably within communities depending on resources, expertise and attitudes to care. General anaesthesia tends to be provided within the hospital setting and this may place limitations on the provision of service. The use of the sedation techniques described have been carried out within the primary care service and therefore minimise such limitation.

The patient's medical condition is inevitably a factor that influences the choice between sedation or general anaesthesia. Sedation offers a less pharmacologically invasive alternative to general anaesthetic which may be safer for those seriously medically compromised. Although ASA III cases may be treated in the primary care setting this should depend on the sedationist's experience and training as well as a careful assessment of the patient's medical condition. One important factor in the choice between general anaesthesia and conscious sedation is the treatment requirement. Multiple and difficult surgical extractions may be inappropriate for treatment using conscious sedation. Similarly, some cases that require extensive restorative treatment may be more appropriately treated under general anaesthesia, enabling treatment to be completed at one visit. In the case of children the first choice of sedation technique may be inhalation sedation and if this proves unsuccessful they are referred for general anaesthesia . However, intranasal and oral sedation with midazolam has been used successfully by the authors for the treatment of children. Other medical/nursing studies[34] and dental research[35] have also shown intranasal midazolam to be a valuable technique in the younger age group. Similarly oral midazolam is used widely in hospital practice as a premedication for children[36], and studies[37] have demonstrated its effective use as an outpatient ambulant technique.

Oral midazolam sedation is by no means new in dentistry, having been described in a study published in 1987[38] in which it compared favourably with intravenous diazepam. Although it has been considered that benzodiazepines are unpredictable when used in children, the potential for the use of these techniques deserves further study.

Factors influencing the choice between GA or sedation as an adjunct to dental treatment:

- availability of the technique – accessible and available
- patient's medical history
- type of dental care required
- patient compliance

Conclusion

Although conscious sedation techniques have been used for some time in both medicine and dentistry, they have not been extensively used in the provision of dental care for people with disability on an ambulant out-patient basis. In this chapter an examination of the literature has been presented, and evidence from clinical practice supports the contention that innovative techniques can be used successfully to meet the specific needs of this patient group and are not simply theoretical alternatives. Such techniques should be used by those who have experience both with providing intravenous sedation and in the management of people with disability.

Within the United Kingdom the practice of sedation in dentistry is regulated in detail by the General Dental Council in its published ethical guidance for dentists[39]. Different regulations apply in different countries. If the use of sedation as presented in this chapter is to be increased there is a clear need for further training in this area. The techniques described are effective and safe methods of providing accessible and acceptable dental care. For the benefit of people with disabilities it is important that those in the dental profession in all countries work together to develop this important area of care.

References

1. Holland T J, O'Mullane D M. The organisation of dental care for groups of mentally handicapped persons. *Community Dent Health* 1990; **7:** 285–293.
2. Report of the Committee on Child Health. *Fit for the future*. London: HMSO, 1976.
3. Worthington L M, Flynn P J, Strunin L. Death in the dental chair: an avoidable catastrophe? *Br J Anaesthesia* 1998; **80:** 131–132.
4. Moore R S, Hobson P. A classification of medically handicapping conditions and the health risks they present in the dental care of children. *J Paed Dent* 1989; **5:** 73–83.
5. Poswillo D. *General anaesthesia, sedation and resuscitation in Dentistry. Report of an Expert Working Party for the Standing Dental Advisory Committee.* London: Department of Health, 1990.
6. Press release and response to reports on general anaesthesia, sedation and resuscitation in dentistry. Department of Health, 1991.
7. *Report of a Working Party on Training in Dental Anaesthesia.* The Royal College of Surgeons of England, 1978.

8. Fukuta O, Braham R L, Yanase H, Atsumi N, Kurosu K. The sedative effect of intranasal midazolam in the dental treatment of patients with mental disabilities. Part I – The effect of a 0.2 mg/kg dose. *J Clin Ped Dent* 1993; **17:** 231–237.

9. Fukuta O, Braham R L, Yanasa H, Kurosu K. The sedative effect of intranasal midazolam in the dental treatment of patients with mental disabilities. Part 2 – Optimal concentrations of intranasal midazolam. *J Clin Paed Dent* 1994; **18:** 259–265.

10. Manford M L M, Roberts G J. Dental treatment in young handicapped patients. An assessment of relative analgaesia as an alternative to general anaesthesia. *Anaesthesia* 1980; **35:** 1157–1168.

11. Blain K M, Hill F J. The use of inhalation sedation and local anaesthesia as an alternative to general anaesthesia for dental extractions in children. *Br Dent J* 1998; **184:** 608–611.

12. Blain K M, Mackie I C. Inhalation sedation: A viable alternative to general anaesthesia? *Dent Update* 1999; **66:** 110–111.

13. Fanning B, Gorby R, Henshaw M, O'Neil A, Treacey C, Vaughan K. Experiences with sedation and restraint during dental treatment in Romania. *J Irish Dent Assoc* 1997; **43:** 22–26.

14. Silver T, Wilson C, Webb M. Evaluation of two doses of oral midazolam as a conscious sedation for physically and neurologically compromised pediatric dental patients. *Ped Dent* 1994; **16:** 350–359.

15. Rosenberg M. Oral Ketamine for deep sedation of difficult-to-manage children who are mentally handicapped: case report. *Ped Dent* 1991; **13:** 221–223.

16. Haney K L, McWhorter A G, Seale N S. An assessment of the success of meperidine and promethazine sedation in medically compromised children. *J Dent Child* 1993; **60:** 288–294.

17. Healey T J. Edmonson H D, Hall N. Sedation for the mentally handicapped patient. *Anaesthesia* 1971; **26:** 308–310.

18. Malamed S F, Gottschalk H W, Mulligan R, Quinn C L. Intravenous sedation for conservative dentistry for disabled patients. *Anaesthesia Prog* 1989; **36:** 140–142.

19. Oei-Lim L B, Vermeulen-Cranch D E, Bouvy Berends E M. Conscious sedation with propofol in dentistry. *Br Dent J* 1991; **170:** 340–344.

20. Oei-Lim L B, Kalkman C J, Makkes P C, Ooms W G, Hoogstraten J. Computer controlled infusion of propofol for conscious sedation in dental treatment. *Br Dent J* 1997; **183:** 204–208.

21. Stephens A J, Sapsford D J, Curzon M E J. Intravenous sedation for handicapped dental patients: a clinical trial of midazolam and propofol. *Br Dent J* 1993; **175:** 20–25.

22. Van der Bijl P, Roelofse J A. Conscious sedation with midazolam in a patient with a spastic nerve muscular disorder-a case report. *Ann Dent* 1994; **53:** 37–38.

23. Van der Bijl P, Roelofse J A. Propofol and midazolam for conscious sedation in a mentally retarded dental patient. *Anaesthesia Prog* 1992; **37:** 37–39.

24. Van der Bijl P, Roelofse J A. Propofol for sedation in a mentally retarded dental patient. *Anaesthesia Prog* 1994; **41:** 81–82.

25. *ABPI Compendium Of Data Sheets.* Data Pharm Publications. London: 1998–9; **11:** 32.

26. *ABPI Compendium Of Data Sheets.* Data Pharm Publications. London: 1998–9; **11:** 1511–152.

27. Bevan J C. Propofol related convulsions. *Can J Anaesthesia* 1993; **40:** 805–809.

28. Dental Practitioners' Formulary. *Prescribing for dental surgeons.* BDA, BMA, RPSGB. London, 1998–2000. pp vii. ·

29. Pickles H. The use of unlicensed drugs. *Br J Health Care Mgt* 1996; **2:** 656–658.

30. Editorial. Unlicensed drug administration. *Anaesthesia* 1995; **50:** 189–190.

31. Cohen M, Gur E, Wertheym E, Shafir R. Intranasal administration of midazolam with a Dinosaur toy (Letter). *Plastic Reconst Surg* 1995; **95:** 421–422.

32. Bjorkman S. Rigemar G, Idvall J. Pharmacokinetics of midazolam given as intranasal spray to adult surgical patients. *Br J Anaesth* 1997; **79:** 575–580.

33. Crevoisier C H, Gieschke R, Heizmann P, Ziegler W H. Pharmacokinetics and pharmacodynamics of midazolam following oral and sublingual administration to healthy volunteers. *Eur Neuropsychopharmacology* 1993; **3:** 2–4.

34. Adrian E R. Intranasal versed: The future of paediatric conscious sedation. *Ped Nurs* 1994; **20:** 287–291.

35. Kaufman E, Davidson E, Sheinkman Z, Magora F. Comparison between intranasal and intravenous midazolam sedation (with or without patient control) in a dental phobia clinic. *J Oral Maxillofacial Surg* 1994; **52:** 840–843.

36. McCluskey A, Meakin G H. Oral administration of midazolam as a premedicant for paediatric day-case anaesthesia. *Anaesthaesia* 1994; **49:** 782–785.

37. Taiwo B, Flowers B, Zoltie N. Reducing children's fear when undergoing painful procedures. *Arch Emerg Med* 1992; **9:** 306–309.

38. O'Boyle C A, Harris D, Barry H, Mccreary C, Bewley A, Fox E. Comparison of midazolam by mouth and diazepam i.v. in outpatient oral surgery. *Br J Anaesth* 1987; **59:** 746–754.

39. *Maintaining standards – guidance to dentists on professional and personal conduct.* London: General Dental Council. Revised November 1998. Amended May 1999.

Chapter 11

Orofacial Dysfunction

Jan Andersson-Norinder and Lotta Sjögreen

The importance of the mouth

Most dentists are focused on the teeth and their diseases. The knowledge about orofacial function and dysfunction is generally poor, which is remarkable since these functions are essential for the quality of life. Why is the orofacial area so important? We use the mouth for breathing, eating and communication. Small children use the mouth as a tool for discovering the world . The orofacial area provides us with valuable sensations like taste, smell, and tactile information. The mouth is also central in non-verbal communication – when we express ourselves with facial mimicry and sounds.

The orofacial anatomy consists of small parts that should fit together as one unit and work together in harmony and balance. Each orofacial structure is adaptable to different functional systems: the airway system, the digestive system, the mimic, and the organ of speech. Neonatal reflexes run the essential orofacial functions from birth. In the older child the orofacial motor function and sensation develops through experience and maturity. Most children can speak and chew well when they are 3- to 4-years old as a result of well developed fine motor function and sensation in the orofacial area. The degree of alertness, motivation, mental capacity, psychological, and medical status influence the orofacial functions. The conditions in the surrounding environment are also of great importance[1] (*Figure1*).

The influence of disabilities on orofacial functions

Anomalies, neurological impairment, different diseases, and trauma usually have an effect on general condition, anatomic structures, motor function, and sensation. This may cause orofacial dysfunction such as sucking and eating problems, speech pathology, impaired facial expression, drooling, bruxism and breathing difficulties in the upper airway system.

The aetiology of orofacial disabilities may be:

* Neurological impairment; congenital, acquired or caused by trauma: for example: cerebral palsy (CP), stroke, Parkinson's disease, multiple sclerosis (MS), amyotrophic lateral sclerosis (ALS)
* Neuromuscular disorders: for example: myotonic dystrophy (DM), Duchenne muscular dystrophy, myasthenia gravis, arthrogryposis multiplexa congenita (AMC), spinal muscular atrophy (SMA)

Figure I

The orofacial complex

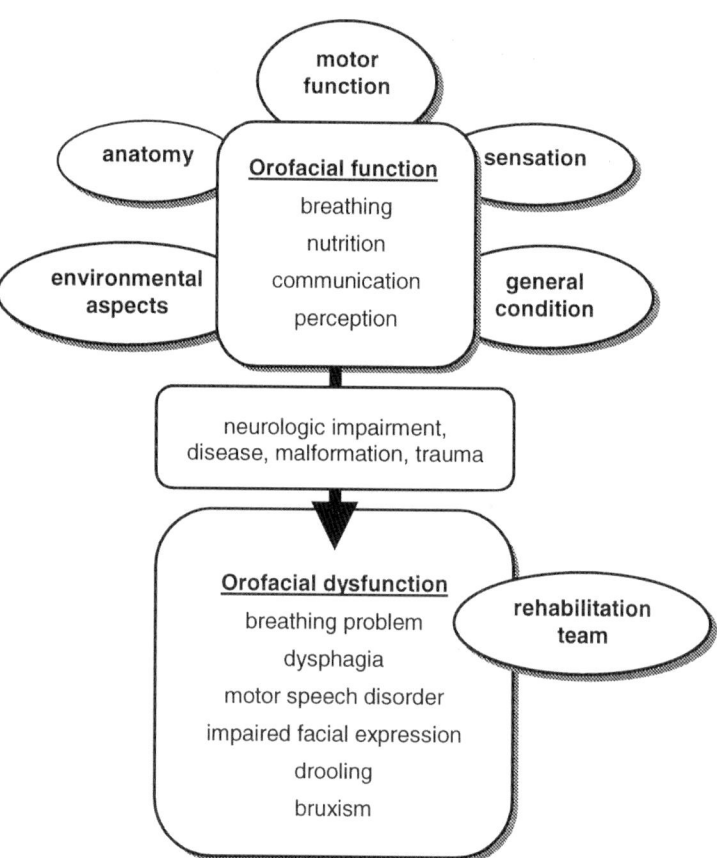

- **Genetic syndromes:** for example: Prader-Willi syndrome (PWS), Down syndrome (DS), Williams syndrome (WS), tuberous sclerosis (TS)
- **Oro-cranio-facial anomalies:** for example: micrognathia, cleft lip and palate, hemifacial microsomia, macroglossia, craniosynostoses

A Swedish survey of 858 individuals with predominantly congenital disorders showed that orofacial dysfunction was very common in this population (*Table 1*). Speech difficulties were found in 52% of the study population, 32% had eating and drinking problems, and 26% were drooling. About 16% had problems with bruxism while 15% were reported to snore[2].

Breathing problems

There are several factors that could cause obstruction in the upper airways and lead to breathing problems: Robin sequence (cleft palate, micrognathia and glossoptosis), hypotonia of the oro-pharyngeal

Table I. Orofacial dysfunction in 858 individuals with different disabilities.

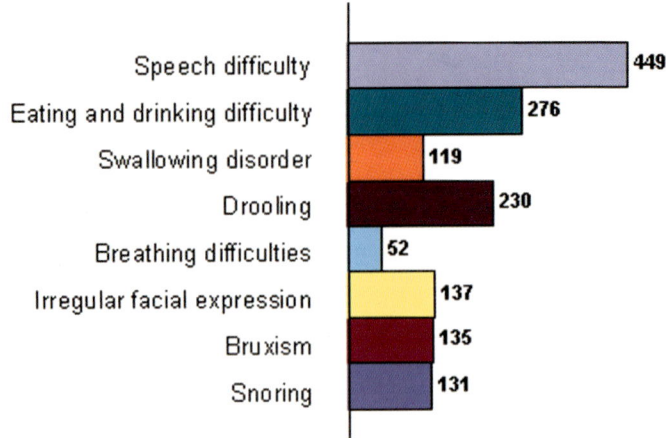

Speech difficulty	449
Eating and drinking difficulty	276
Swallowing disorder	119
Drooling	230
Breathing difficulties	52
Irregular facial expression	137
Bruxism	135
Snoring	131

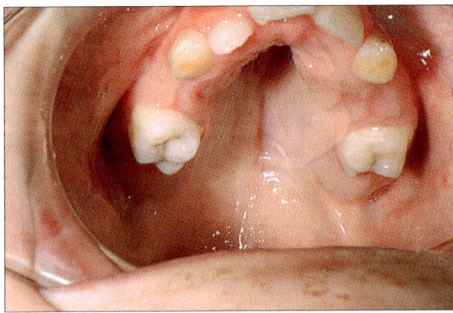

Figure 2
High vaulted palates lead to sleep apnoea

muscles, hypertrophied tonsils and adenoid tissue, choanal atresia, hypoplasia of the jaws, or a high and narrow palate. Some of these symptoms are risk factors for sleep apnoea and they are common among people with disabilities. The dentist should be aware of these risks and refer the patient to an ENT specialist if sleep apnoea is suspected. Orthodontic analysis and treatment is also indicated in most cases. As an example, an extremely high and narrow palate is one of the classic signs in Sotos syndrome. Sleep apnoea is over-represented among these patients and mouth breathing is very common (*Figure 2*).

Common causes of breathing problems:

- Robin sequence
- hypotonia
- enlarged tonsils and adenoids
- choanal atresia
- jaw hypoplasia

- high vaulted palate
- macroglossia

Dysphagia/eating problems

Oral motor impairment or cranio-facial anomalies may cause sucking problems in infancy. However, the feeding abilities are, of course, also very dependent upon the general condition of the child. Congenital heart defects, breathing difficulties as well as gastrointestinal problems are common reasons for feeding disorders. Impaired oral motor function and weak muscles will cause chewing problems and affect swallowing. Dysfunction in the pharyngeal phase of swallowing could cause aspiration of food into the airways and thus become life threatening[3]. Dental problems, severe malocclusion, and impaired jaw opening are other reasons for eating disorders where the dentist must be responsible for the treatment.

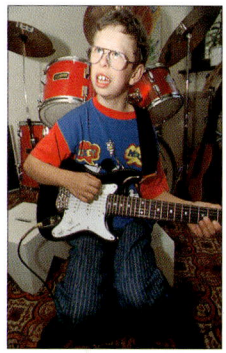

"Johan has two kinds of disabilities, Williams syndrome and Autism. Williams syndrome is a very rare condition and is caused by a micro-deletion on chromosome 7. The syndrome leads to mental retardation with a very special appearance and behaviour problems. Most children with Williams syndrome have sucking problems. Thus, Johan was not breastfed as an infant. Instead, he had to be fed with a bottle with an enlarged hole. Children with Williams syndrome also have chewing and swallowing problems. Johan was almost three years old when he was able to eat semisolid food. The autism and the difficulties when encountering new tastes and consistencies did not make it easier. Gradually, Johan has been trained to accept new dishes.

Johan uses his tongue when chewing and not so much his teeth. His favourite foods are porridge, potatoes and bananas, which are easy to chew.

Today, at nine years old he can, with some difficulties, eat well-cut food and vegetables but he is still not very fond of this food.

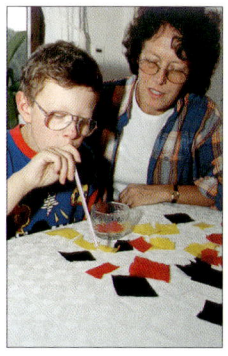

In order to help Johan we have trained his oral muscles with sucking and blowing exercises and the last year he has also been training with an oral screen. By orthodontic treatment and daily training we hope that Johan will have a normalised eating behaviour as a grown up."
(A letter from Maria, Johan's mother)

Williams syndrome is a condition where feeding and eating problems are common (*Table 2*). The patients often have congenital heart defects, oral motor impairment, malocclusion, and a hypersensitive mouth.

Common causes of feeding/eating problems:
- craniofacial anomalies

107

Table 2. The frequency of eating problems in 56 individuals with Williams syndrome

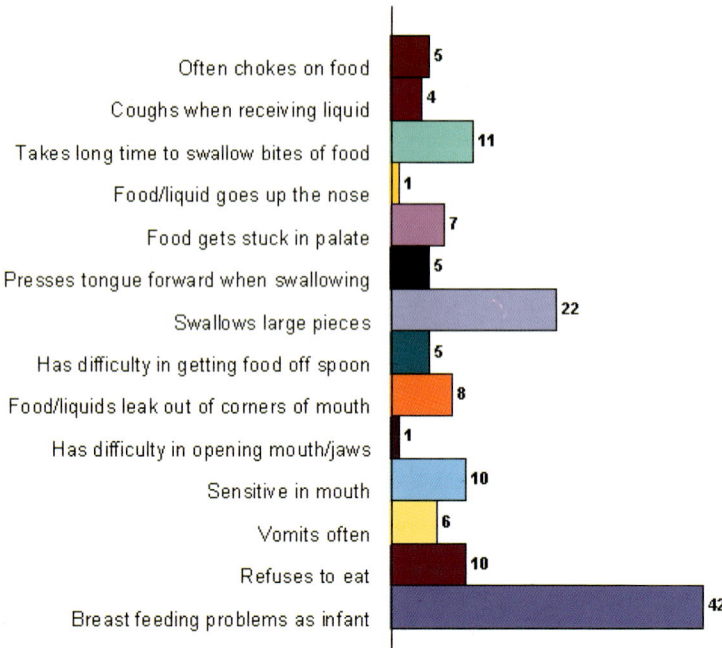

Often chokes on food	5
Coughs when receiving liquid	4
Takes long time to swallow bites of food	11
Food/liquid goes up the nose	1
Food gets stuck in palate	7
Presses tongue forward when swallowing	5
Swallows large pieces	22
Has difficulty in getting food off spoon	5
Food/liquids leak out of corners of mouth	8
Has difficulty in opening mouth/jaws	1
Sensitive in mouth	10
Vomits often	6
Refuses to eat	10
Breast feeding problems as infant	42

- breathing difficulties
- congenital heart defects
- impaired oral motor function
- swallowing dysfunction
- dental anomalies
- limited mouth opening

Motor speech disorders

Articulation demands very fine motor control and is, therefore, sensitive to oral motor impairment and deviant anatomic structures. On the other hand, the ability to compensate for articulation difficulties is often surprisingly good. Neurological impairment could lead to dysarthria or anarthria. Malocclusion or minor oral motor dysfunctions could often explain minor articulation problems (dyslalia). Apraxia of speech is an impaired ability, in the absence of obvious muscular disturbance of the speech mechanism, to voluntarily carry out the expected motor gestures and programming of gestures needed for the articulation of speech. This condition is seen in both congenital and acquired disorders and its true background is not yet fully understood. Stuttering could be characterised as a speech rhythm disorder. The aetiology of stuttering is not known[4]. There seems to be an over representation of stuttering in some genetic disorders, for instance Down syndrome and Tourette's syndrome.

Common speech disorders in disabled people:
- Dysarthria/anarthria – impaired articulation
- Dyslalia – minor articulation problems
- Apraxia – failure to articulate speech
- Stuttering

Communication disorders are common in children and adults with different disabilities and is often caused by a combination of articulation, language, and pragmatic difficulties. Hearing is of course also vital for communication.

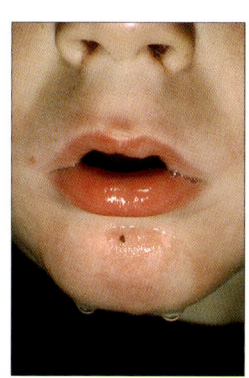

Figure 3

The typical facies of a child with a drooling problem

Drooling

The cause of drooling is very seldom hyper-salivation. Even in Parkinson's disease, where hyper-salivation has often been reported, it has not been validated. Perhaps the drooling problems are caused by dysphagia, which is also common in Parkinson's disease. The general condition of the person and any medical treatment are very important factors influencing drooling. Poor lip closure, malocclusion, impaired motility in the tongue, and poor stability in the neck are other important factors (*Figure 3*). Oral habits, that are common in many neurological diseases and genetic syndromes, also cause drooling. In a survey in Sweden of 979 individuals with different disabilities, 346 had drooling of which 84 had slight drooling, 116 moderate, 80 profuse, and 43 very profuse (*Table 3*)[2]. It should be pointed out that drooling also affects the quality of life as it is not seen as acceptable in normal social life.

Table 3. The frequence of drooling in 979 individuals with different disabilities

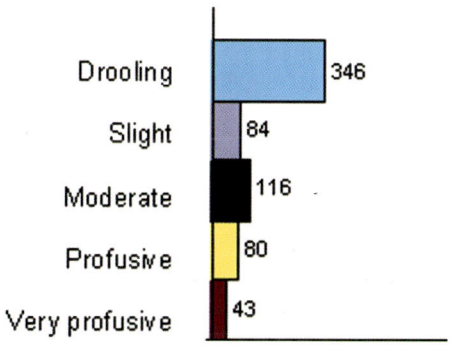

Drooling	346
Slight	84
Moderate	116
Profusive	80
Very profusive	43

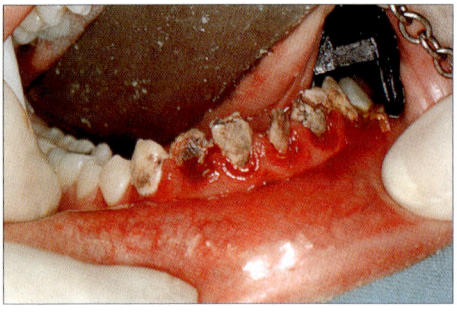

Figure 4

Dental caries as a consequence of xerostomia in a patient who had salivary glands excised because of excessive drooling

Causes of drooling:

- Dysphagia
- Poor lip seal
- Malocclusion
- Impaired soft tissue motility
- Poor neck stability
- Oral habits

The treatment of drooling could be physiologic, surgical or pharmacological[5]. Physiotherapy with an oral screen strengthens the peri-oral muscles and improves lip closure. Further, training with an oral screen also affects swallowing by strengthening the buccinator muscles and the upper constrictor muscles in the pharynx ("the buccinator mechanism"). Orthodontic treatment, and sometimes orthognatic surgery, is indicated to create optimal inter-maxillary relations in order to facilitate lip closure. Different surgical approaches have been advocated for the control of drooling. The saliva production can be reduced by excision of salivary glands or the salivary gland ducts can be posteriorly re-routed. Another surgical method is sectioning the parasympathetic supply to the salivary glands. If surgery results in xerostomia, preventive dental strategies/treatments should be given high priority since these patients are at high risk of developing dental caries (*Figure 4*). Treatment with anticholinergic drugs, e.g. hyoscine patches, is effective but can produce unacceptable side effects (*Figures 5a and 5b*).

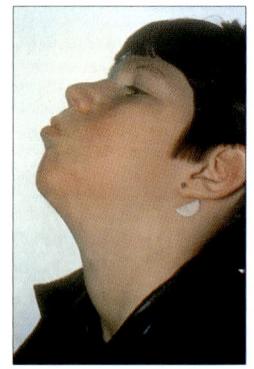

Figure 5a

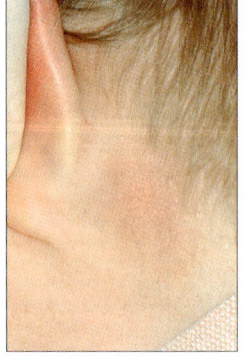

Figure 5b

Figure 6

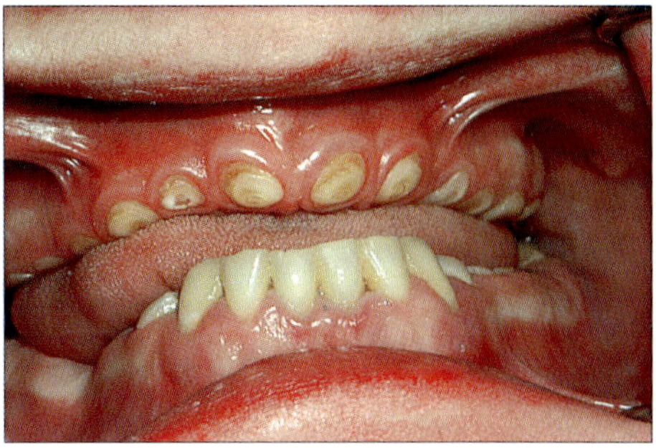

Treatment options for drooling:
- Physiotherapy
- Oral motor appliances
- Orthodontic treatment
- Salivary gland surgery
- Nerve resection
- Drugs
- Orthognathic surgery

Bruxism

Grinding and clenching may lead to wear of teeth. Among individuals with neurological impairment tooth wear could be very severe (*Figure 6*). The worst form, daytime bruxism, also results in great social problems because of noise. The reason for this daytime bruxism is not known. However, many of these individuals are severely mentally retarded, often autistic, and have no means of communication. There are theories that bruxism could be a self-destructing activity. It has also been suggested that bruxism stimulates neurological activities resulting in light and sound sensations perceived as positive by the individual. Another theory is that bruxism can stimulate the production of endorphins. Whatever the cause, it is very important to find methods to reduce bruxism and protect the teeth. Orofacial massage for relaxation combined with soft and hard acrylic splints have been used for treatment but this is an area for further research.

Rehabilitation

Different professionals are generally involved in the assessment, evaluation, and treatment of the complex orofacial dysfunctions detailed above. Ideally, these professionals work together in a team making it possible to analyse the dysfunction in a holistic perspective and make a treatment plan. The dentist has an important role to play in this team, not only to care for the oral health but also to improve orofacial function by means of orthodontic treatment, orthognatic surgery,

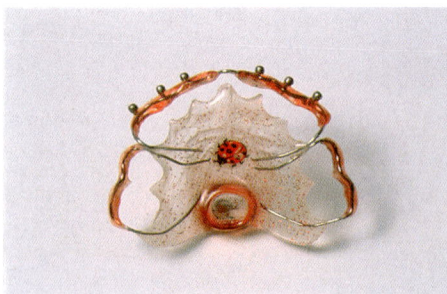

Figure 7
Removable appliance for intraoral stimulation

Figure 8
Oral screens for lip training

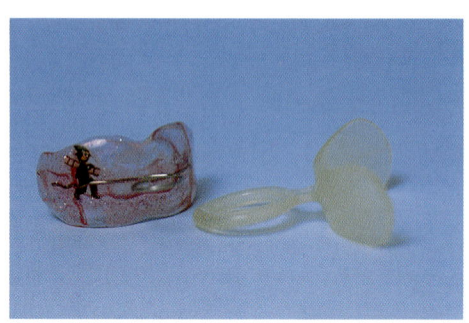

prosthethics, and oral motor training. Oral motor treatment is preferably planned together with speech therapists and physiotherapists.

New methods for orofacial therapy are constantly developing but there is a need for better instruments to evaluate the effects of training and treatment. Orofacial massage is used to affect the muscle tone and to improve mobility through sensory-motor stimulation. Intra-oral massage can stimulate the sucking reflex and prevent hypersensitivity in the mouth in connection with tube feeding. Exercises for lips, tongue and chewing muscles could strengthen the muscles and improve motility. Sometimes an intra-oral appliance, like a palatal plate (*Figure 7*) or an oral screen (*Figure 8*), could be effective in oral motor training. The vibrations from an electrical toothbrush give intense tactile sensations and could be used for stimulation of the muscles inside and outside the mouth. In orofacial rehabilitation it is important to find activities in daily life that support orofacial function e.g. mouth toys, straw sucking, chewing gum, blowing instruments, mashed or liquidised food.

Many patients with orofacial dysfunctions require aids for feeding, eating, drinking, and oral motor training. Spoons for feeding should be in plastic material as metal spoons may cause wear of the teeth (*Figures 9 and 10*). To avoid extension of the neck when drinking a cut-out cup can be use (*Figure 11*). A palatal plate with a movable ring on a metal bar could be an aid to improve the lateral tongue movements (*Figure 12*).

Figures 9 and 10

Tooth wear as a consequence of using a metal spoon

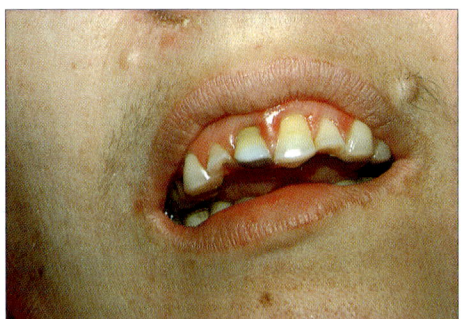

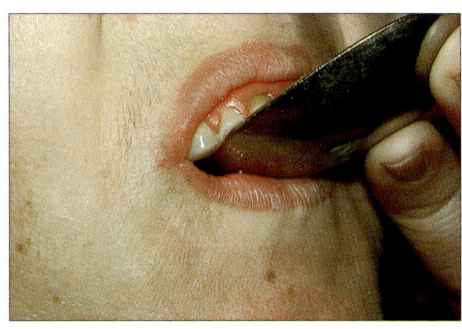

Figure 11

Use of a cut-out cup to prevent neck extension

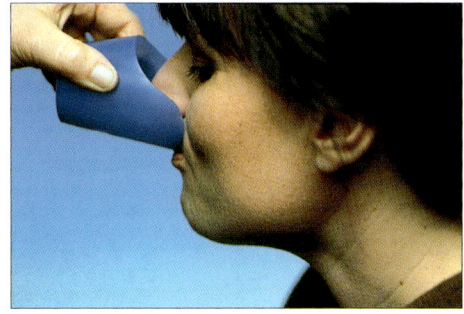

Figure 12

An appliance design to improve lateral tongue movements

Conclusion

If you are to be successful in treatment of orofacial dysfunction it is necessary to work together with other professionals. Thus, the dentist must be a member of the rehabilitation team. There is an urgent need to increase knowledge about orofacial rehabilitation for people with disabilities and new methods for treatment must be developed and evaluated. This will lead to better care and will have great influence on the quality of life for people with disabilities.

References

1. Castillo Morales R, Haberstock B, Brondo J. *Die orofacial regulationsterapi*. 1991.
2. Mun-H-Center database. 1999.
3. Andersson J C, Bridsky L. *Pediatric Swallowing and Feeding*. 1999.
4. Russel J L. *Childhood Motor Speech Disability*. 1992.
5. Finkelstein D M, Chrysdale W S. Evaluation and management of the drooling patient. *J Otolaryngology* 1992; **21**: 414–417.

Chapter 12

Community Dental Programmes

Peter King

Introduction

Community dental health programmes for patients with special needs exist in urban and rural centres throughout the world. They address the barriers to accessing dental care experienced by people with disabilities. However, the range of services offered by different community dental health programmes, their administration and their support varies enormously.

Factors contributing to these variations include:

- Which groups of people with disabilities are targeted by the service
- What structures are currently in place in the community to educate, employ and house people with disabilities
- Demographics
- Geography
- Available funding
- Available expertise

Establishing a community dental health programme that meets the needs of people with disabilities in a given population requires careful planning. In other words, for people with disabilities, the barriers to accessing dental care in that population needs to be defined; priorities, goals and objectives established; and a method of implementation determined[1].

While the structure of community dental health programmes will vary, there are several characteristics of a community dental health service for people with disabilities that are vital to providing a successful, comprehensive service[2].

Characteristics of community dental health programmes

1. Clear guidelines regarding who can access the service

The inclusion of all groups of people with disability in a community dental health service or the exclusion of some groups will be contingent on the available resources, the demographics of the community, available expertise and the existing oral health services available to each of the groups. Furthermore, within each of these groups of disability the range of inability to access existing dental services varies. Strict guidelines should exist regarding who can access a community dental health service to ensure that funds allocated to community dental health programmes for people with disabilities reaches those people with disabilities who have the greatest need for a specialised service.

The range of people with disabilities that have been included in community dental health programmes include:

- people with intellectual disabilities;
- people with physical disabilities;
- people with mental illness;
- frail and functionally dependent elderly.

2. Staff Trained in Special Care Dentistry

Many dentists report low confidence in their ability to manage patients with special needs[3]. Furthermore, there is little or no training of special care dentistry in many oral health undergraduate programmes. Members of a community dental health team need to understand modifying factors which exist that influence the management and treatment planning for people with disabilities.

Modifying factors include:

- Difficulty removing plaque
- Difficulty communicating needs
- A reliance on carers
- Poor clearance of foodstuff from the oral cavity
- Greater use of medications that cause xerostomia
- Congenital abnormalities that may affect oro-motor function, saliva, dental occlusion and dental structures
- A higher risk of malnutrition
- A greater need for a range of sedation techniques for routine dental care
- A need for practitioners who are skilled at modifying challenging behaviours in the dental setting to minimise the use of sedation.

Orientation programmes, in-service training and a staff development strategy is required that provides training in the oral health management of people with disabilities.

3. Liaison Person

Community dental health programmes interact with a wide range of individuals and organisations. People with disabilities, their carers, families, teachers, medical personnel and institutional bodies that co-ordinate education, housing and employment for people with disabilities will all have an interest in a community dental health pro-gramme for people with disabilities.

The liaison person's role is to facilitate good communication between the community dental health programme and the community it serves.

Responsibilities of the liaison person will include:

- Disseminating information to interested parties about the services provided by the unit
- Co-ordinating available community supported transport to carry patients to and from dental appointments
- Preparing an organisation for the arrival of a dental team for screen-ing or domiciliary care to ensure that the needs of the dental team and the requirements of the organisation being visited are each honoured.
- Maintaining systems that ensure patients are reviewed appropriately.

4. Portable Equipment

When resources are limited and the demand is great, it is important to have effective screening programmes that can ensure people with disabilities are regularly examined and that their needs can be assessed and prioritised. By providing screening programmes in a location outside of the dental clinical setting, some of the fears associated with a dental visit are also addressed. The location of screening programmes may include institutions, sheltered workshops, schools for people with disabilities, activity centres for people with disabilities and nursing homes.

The availability of portable equipment enables a community dental health programme to:

- screen groups of patients
- provide treatment in less threatening settings
- provide treatment to homebound patients
- extend an urban special care service into rural areas

Portable equipment also ensures that people, who are truly homebound, can access dental care. There is a large range of portable equipment available for the restorative management of patients in a non-clinical setting (Chapter 14).

Furthermore, the expertise that is required by a community dental health team and the associated costs involved often leaves rural areas without a specialised facility for people with disabilities. Portable equipment opens the possibility of a highly experienced dental team in urban areas, providing services to people with disabilities in rural areas on a seasonal basis[4].

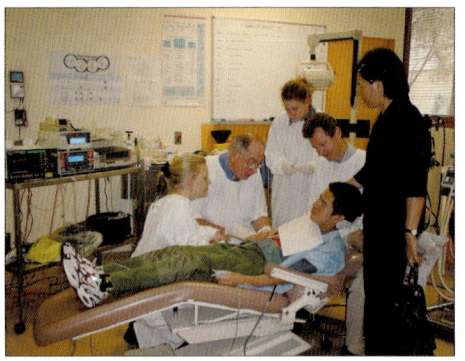

Figure 1

Intravenous sedation during a community programme

5. Flexibility

A community dental health service must accept that the likelihood of patients arriving late and needing to change appointments is greater than in other disciplines of dentistry. The co-ordination of carers, specialised transport needs and the greater incidence of illness in people with disabilities makes the need for flexibility in a community dental service paramount. There is also a greater chance that appointments, once attended, will be interrupted or need an extension of time to accommodate the management of challenging behaviours.

Allowing flexibility and at the same time ensuring productivity is a challenging task. A team approach to managing patients is essential to meet each of these requirements.

6. Sedation

The management of challenging behaviour requires the availability of a range of sedation (*Figure 1*). While intravenous and general anaesthetic facilities are often available for oral surgery procedures, the availability of these services for periodontal care and conservative restorative care of people with disabilities is more frequently scarce. However, without these services, the range of treatment options available is limited.

7. Inter-disciplinary support

Oral health is an integral part of general health. The oral health practitioner will encounter dental problems that will require the opinion and treatment of medical practitioners. For example, the prevalence of reflux is higher in people with disabilities than in the general community[5]. The observation of dental erosion can play an important role in identifying reflux or rumination behaviour in a person with a disability and subsequent referral and management by a gastroenterologist is essential (*Figures 2–5*). While it is not essential to have medical support

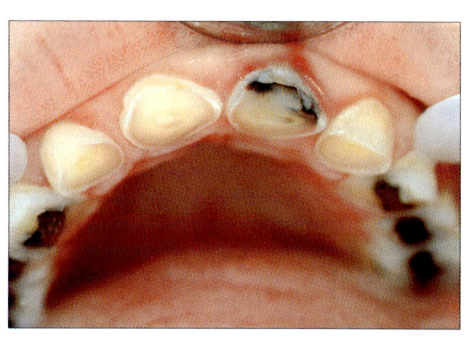

Figure 2

Advanced tooth tissue loss as a consequence of gastro-oesophageal reflux in a patient with cerebral palsy

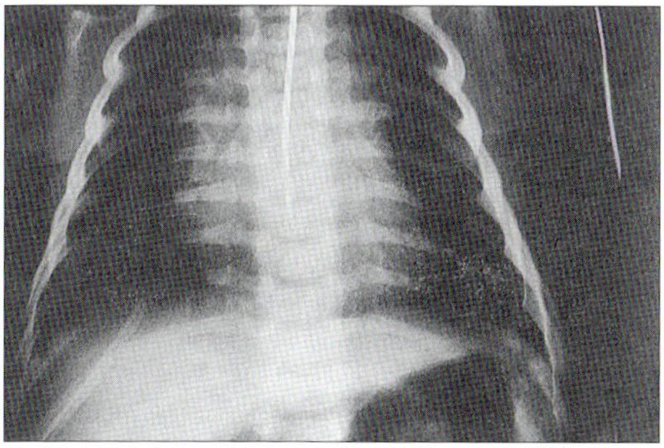

Figure 3

Positioning of an intra-oesophageal pH probe to determine the presence of reflux

Figure 4

The pH tracing obtained from a patient with gastro-oesophageal reflux - for much of the monitoring period the pH was well below the critical value of 4

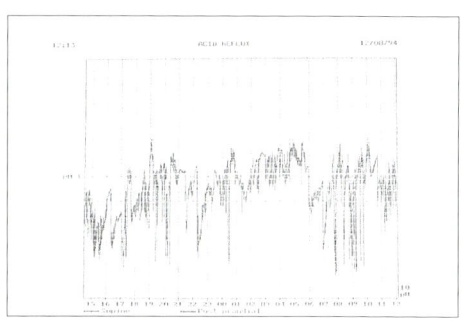

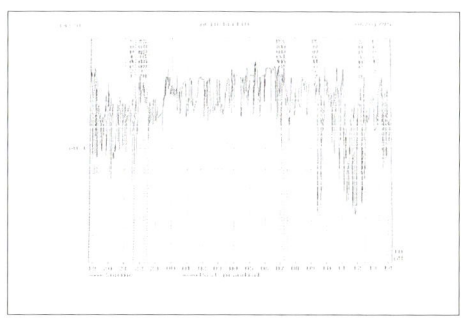

Figure 5

A similar trace to that recorded in Figure 4 in a patient with reflux that has been treated with an appropriate drug. For much of the monitoring period the pH is well above the critical value apart from periods when the patient is supine.

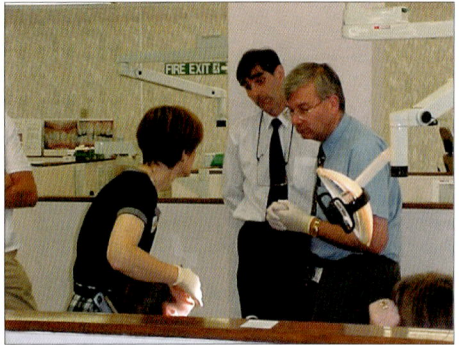

Figure 6

Interdisciplinary working is essential for the optimal management of patients with disabilities

on site, a system of referral and management needs to be established.

The risks and side effects of general anaesthetic and intravenous sedation also highlight the need for community dental health programmes to have medical support and in many countries it is mandatory for general anaesthesia for dentistry to be administered only in hospitals with appropriate medical back-up.

The management of patients' oral health needs requires the involvement of all the specialities of dentistry to ensure that a full range of services are available to people with disabilities.

The community dental health unit will need to foster links with:

- oral surgeons
- periodontists
- prosthdontists
- orthodontists

Links with allied health professionals are also essential. Findings from an oral health assessment may lead to referral to speech pathologists, occupational therapists, physiotherapists and psychologists. For example, inter-disciplinary clinics exist throughout the world for the management of poor saliva control. Providing an inter- disciplinary clinic to treat sialorrhoea has significant advantages[6]. Firstly, it allows the patient to be informed of the surgical approach, behavioural approach, medications and intra-oral appliances (*Figure 6*) that are used in differing circumstances to treat sialhorrea. Secondly, it allows the dentist, speech pathologist, physician and therapist to interact and consider the most appropriate management of each patient. People with disabilities frequently consult a variety of health professionals in relation to any one problem and they are often left to make decisions about their treatment at the end of an exhausting search for information. Inter-disciplinary clinics puts the emphasis on the professionals to weigh up the advantages and disadvantages of different strategies to manage a particular problem and to give information to the patient in a concise efficient manner. Inter-disciplinary teams allow the client and carer to be informed about all the options available to manage a particular problem.

8. Oral health promotion

Improving the oral health behaviours of people with disabilities and their carers is a crucial activity of community dental health programmes. Numerous programmes have been established for carers of people with mental illness[7], intellectual disabilities[8], and the functionally dependent elderly[9,10]. They have proved to be effective tools in improving oral health behaviours of caregivers. Other programmes focusing on improving the skills of people with disabilities at plaque removal have also proven to be effective[11].

Oral health promotional activities need to be focused on specific client or carer groups, have defined outcomes and be carefully evaluated.

9. Multiple objectives

Successful community dental health programmes usually have multiple objectives which include university teaching and research[2]. Scholarship required for these activities generates knowledge that is useful to all aspects of a community dental health programme.

10. Attention to occupational health and safety

While most health services are acutely aware of the significance of occupational health and safety, the community dental health service has some unique factors to consider when establishing their occupational health and safety policies.

Health and safety issues related to community health programmes:

- management of aggressive behaviour
- the transfer of patients from wheelchairs and beds
- carrying and setting up portable equipment at non clinical locations
- infection control in non clinical settings

References

1. Jong A W. *Community Dental Health.* 3rd edition. Mosby. 225–229.
2. Burtner A P, Dicks J L. Providing oral health care to individuals with severe disabilities residing in the community: Alternative care delivery systems. *Spec Care Dent* 1994; **14:** 188–192.
3. Oliver C H, Nunn J H. The accessibility of dental treatment to adults with physical disabilities in northeast England. *Spec Care Dent* 1996; **16:** 204–209.
4. Glassman P, Miller C E, Leckowick J. A dental school's role in developing rural, community-based,

dental care delivery system for individuals with developmental disabilities. *Spec Care Dent* 1996; **16:** 188–193.

5. Lennox N. *People with developmental and intellectual disabilities*. Therapeutic Guidelines Ltd.: Melbourne, 1999, 51–53.

6. Hussein I, Kershaw A E, Tahmassebi J F et al. The management of drooling in children and patients with mental and physical disabilities: a review of the literature. *Int J Paed Dent* 1998; **8:** 3–11.

7. Chalmers J, Kingsford Smith D, Knute D C. A Multidisciplinary dental program for community living adults with chronic mental illness. *Spec Care Dent* 1998; **18:** 194–201.

8. Glassman P, Miller C, Wozniak T, Jones C. A preventive dentistry training program for caretakers of people with disabilities residing in the community. *Spec Care Dent* 1994; **14:** 137–143.

9. Frenkel H. A health education intervention to improve the oral health of institutional elderly people: a randomised controlled trial. PhD thesis. Faculty of Dentistry, University of Bristol, 1998.

10. King P. A dental health education program for carers of elderly people in nursing homes. Masters thesis. Faculty of Dentistry, University of Sydney, 1993.

11. Shapira J, Stabholz A. A Comprehensive 30-month preventive dental health program in a pre-adolescent population with Down's Syndrome: A longitudinal study. *Spec Care Dent* 1996; **16:** 33–37.

Chapter 13

Hospital Dentistry

Clive Friedman

Introduction

A hospital dental service is an essential service for the provision of comprehensive oral health care within the hospital environment. The scope of this service will differ dependant on the nature and mission of the hospital and the needs of the community[1,2].

Essential services of hospital based dentistry:

- **Operating room management** of paediatric, 'special needs', dental and oral and maxillofacial surgical patients is often the only dental treatment provided in a hospital.
- **Developmentally challenged and medically compromised people**, due to the unique nature and challenge posed in their management, the hospital environment is often the safest and most reasonable way to provide dental treatment. This is especially the case when no other resources are available in the community. Frequently the operating room is the only option for completion of restorative treatment or even an examination. Individuals who fall into PARS Category III–V (table 3, Chapter 6) are ideal candidates for a hospital dental service.
- **Consulting services for medical disciplines** Dentists provide and act on the interdisciplinary teams treating patients with multiple problems such as transplant, haemophiliac, oncologic and cranio-facial patients.
- **Partner with medical colleagues** in the management of emergency room and trauma patients.
- **Teaching and research** could be included dependant on the nature of the hospital but would be better classified as associated services not essential to the operation of a hospital based dental clinic.

Many types of patients may be and indeed are treated in a hospital clinic but they could just as easily be treated in a community setting. This chapter will concentrate on persons with disabilities treated in a hospital setting.

History and current political climate

Hospital Dentistry is a community-based resource. As such, Hospital Dentistry at least in North America, is currently going through variations of changing paradigms and budgetary upheavals[3,4]. In days when funding was adequate, dental departments within hospitals had the luxury of being able to treat a plethora of difficult and 'special needs' patients without recourse to heavily scrutinised, evidence-based and overly justified financial responsibility. Many indigent, (homeless, poor, disabled) have turned to hospital departments as primary care facilities. This pool of patients was in addition to the traditional patient who presented with chronic illness, or required the hospital setting due to medically adjunctive needs. As health care dollars have become scarce, hospitals are becoming increasingly more cost conscious. Dental departments within hospitals are now being required to be revenue neutral or profit-making centres. Thus, the traditional roles of serving the indigent and the medically compromised dental patient have to be incorporated into different philosophical processes. The treatment of these patient populations are costly and do not generate funds for departments. In the past, funding for these services have come from within global hospital budgets or other government programmes.

Today payment vehicles for funding dental treatment may include[5]:

- **Government funding** – either on a national health basis or for specific target populations. This would be dependant on the prevailing economic philosophy of a country. This is the likely source of funding for most hospital dental departments in the world.
- **Social Service or Welfare** – Dependant on prevailing country economic system.
- **Service Organisations** – The Excella Grotto, a division of the Masons, specifically support dentistry for children with disabilities. Only 3 divisions currently operate in Canada, many more are active in the United States. Funding from Grotto will often cover dental needs that are not covered by normal programmes such as orthodontics. The Shriners, also a division of the Masons, support burn units across North America.
- **Charitable Foundations** – for example, the Robert Wood Johnson Foundation – awarded up to 10 million in grants to hospitals across the United States to increase availability of dental care to indigent and medically compromised people[6].
- **Private Insurance Carriers**
- **Individual Patient responsibility**. The percentage of the population covering dental costs through the last two means would also be heavily country dependant.

In order to achieve revenue neutrality dental departments in hospitals in North America today are finding many innovative solutions in order to survive. These include but are not limited to:

- **Downsizing**: Providing only minimal and essential care on site. This solution requires the establishment of outpatient clinics that are capable of providing mostly outpatient care with general anaesthesia facilities, to PARS and ASA I, II, and III patients.

- **Centralisation of specialty clinics**: Centralising clinics such as cleft palate clinics to only one hospital in a state/province instead of having multiple centres, ostensibly creating different centres of excellence.
- **Establishing well patient clinics:** Regular private practice care is being provided within the hospital setting to patients that could have this treatment done in the community. This population is more likely to generate revenue that can then be used to offset the costs of the more difficult-to-care-for patient. (The cost of providing care within the hospital setting is however much more expensive, due to the subsidisation of space by hospitals).
- **In-hospital dental care programmes**: Dental care is provided to hospital employees.
- **Outreach programmes**: The hospital dentists are providing care and programmes in a variety of community settings. These settings such as homes for elderly people often have little or no access to good care and innovative dental departments are supplementing their budgets by providing this care.
- **Medically adjunctive care**: (Medically necessary oral health care that is a direct result of, or has a direct impact on, an underlying medical condition and /or its resulting therapy.) Medically necessary oral health care is integral to comprehensive treatment to ensure optimum health care outcomes. It can potentially reduce health care expenditures for treatment of costly complications for example, heart defects, head and neck radiation, developmental disabilities. As more of this type of information is gathered the costs can more easily be accrued to the overall health budget.

Role of the hospital in care for persons with disability

Recent trends in many of the developing countries to normalisation (the process whereby persons with disabilities are being encouraged to live in as normal an environment as possible within their communities with local support, rather than living in institutions) has resulted in large numbers of people entering the community without the support that they previously enjoyed in the institutions (see Chapter15). As a result, the demography of the population is rapidly changing. This includes psychiatric, as well as moderately and profoundly disabled individuals. There are 170 million individuals in the world with mental retardation, very few have access to adequate dental care within their communities[3]. Even within the United States the data collected on more than two thousand Special Olympic athletes screened in 1998 identified that 35% of the athletes were in need of care[7]. Remembering that athletes competing in special Olympics would be relatively high functioning individuals, the percentage of individuals needing care among the total special needs population would be that much greater. The reasons for this are varied. They include:

- **Limited funding** available for this population[3].
- **Inadequate education of students** within dental schools. In both a 1993 and 1998 survey of US and Canadian dental schools, the average number of lecture hours devoted to care for patients with special needs was less than 13. Clinical instruction constituted only 0–5% of a student's time. Disappointingly there was even a decrease from the 1993 to the 1998 survey[8,9].
- **Difficulty of management**[10]
- **Behavioural disturbance** of private practice environment
- **A low profile area** of the dental profession. In a recent editorial Fenton describes how many hospitals not only do not have facilities to provide comprehensive treatment but no interest is shown to establish them either[11].

The needs for specialty clinics within hospitals where persons can be referred and treated are becoming important community resources in obtaining care. Further, paediatric dentists have traditionally taken care of many individuals with special needs. The life span of this population is increasing with better medical health. Many more individuals are reaching ages where paediatric dentists are no longer willing to treat, but have nowhere to refer this growing population. Thus clinics, such as adult disabilities clinics, are being established within hospital settings or within institutions. Many dental departments already have clinics that treat children with special needs. These clinics act as teaching environments for paediatric dentists, as well as university students and general practice residencies. The specific dental care provided within the hospital setting should be no different than that being provided within the community or in a private practice setting. The only difference is the environment; which has an accumulation of individuals with the appropriate knowledge base whereby all the needs of the person with the disability can be taken care of. Within such clinics particular emphasis can be placed on support and training.

Patient selection criteria

This would be dependant on the nature of the funding base for a particular hospital department. The patients seen at the special needs clinic in London, Ontario are all patients that have been unable to obtain care from dentists within the community.

Oral and dental care

Emphasis is placed on preventive programming and home care.

The Health History Form (Form 1)

Apart from the normal questions in such a history note the specific questions regarding issues such as self help skills and home care. The skill survey and preventive programme form (*Form 2*) evaluates the specific skill of a patient and provides for individualised programme development and follow up. This form can be used in the clinic or sent home with the care giver or parent as an adjunct in obtaining good daily oral care.

Treatment options

Within the hospital environment a plethora of treatment options are available in the provision of care. These include desensitisation, hypnosis, protective support, sedation and both in- and out-patient general anaesthesia.

Staffing requirements

Personnel working on a continual basis with persons with special needs, require specific training in dealing with this patient group. A variety of different training modules have been developed which help in this training programme. These modules address the training of both dental staff as well as direct care staff[12-16].

Specialty clinics and teams

Due to the collection of many different specialties within the hospital setting it is a unique environment for the creation of specialty clinics and interdisciplinary teams in order to provide a combined treatment approach to those who have multiple and difficult requirements. The hospital setting itself is not essential for the establishment of these teams; however, in many countries, this is where they traditionally find themselves.

Examples of hospital-led interdisciplinary teams:

- Craniofacial anomalies
- Feeding disorders
- Drooling clinics
- Cancer rehabilitation
- Sleep apnoea laboratories
- Cleft palate teams (*addendum 1*)

Oral health teams consisting of periodontics, prosthodontics, paediatric, orthodontics and other medical specialties as required are members of these teams and are only limited by the dental department and accessibility to such specialties. A detailed example of the protocol used for cleft palate patients at the Children's Hospital, Calgary,

Alberta can be seen in *addendum 1*[17]. It clearly identifies how the numerous specialties and departments within a hospital team interact at different ages of the child[18].

"Team" evaluations of hospital patients often require dental input and certain medical protocols require routine dental evaluations. Thus dentists may be involved in patient services in areas such as:

* In patient consultations
* Cancer clinics
* Haemophiliac clinics
* Cardiac clinics (Protocol in *addendum 2*)
* Organ transplant clinics (Protocol for bone marrow transplants in *addendum 3*)[18]

Administrative organisation and hospital privileges

In order to practice within a hospital setting requirements differ according to country, state and prevailing dental politics within different countries. In the US for example, following a specific credentialing process and appointment to medical dental staff, dentists are required to fulfil certain responsibilities. These may include patient care within the approved clinical privileges, participation in emergency room call, appropriate completion of records, and compliance with the rules and regulations of the particular hospital[1,2,4].

In Canada, for example, remote areas are far less stringent on the credentials required for hospital admittance than big cities or university towns. However, in big cities even as a specialist with appropriate training and credentials it may be impossible to obtain privileges. (Required permission to work within the hospital environment). Economics and local politics often play a big role in these determinations.

In third world countries it is very similar to the rural or remote areas of Canada where the mere willingness to work in the hospital affords one the opportunity of being able to work. In most instances of this nature the only service available is often oral surgery and not restorative dentistry. Countries like Mexico have different problems in that materials are difficult or expensive to obtain and the culture perceives the need for dental care for persons with disability very differently. To many it is an embarrassment to even bring such a child for care.

Sedation and general anaesthesia

Provision of sedation within a hospital setting

Access. Some hospitals have specific operating rooms designated to dentistry where the full spectrum of materials and instruments are available to provide comprehensive care. In others one is required to take ones own equipment to the hospital. Many companies have created

London Health Sciences Centre
Department of Dentistry, Special Needs Clinic

Confidential Medical/Dental History

PIN# _____

Name:_____Birth date(D/M/Y):_____
     (Last Name)   (First Name)

Address:_____

City:_____Postal Code:_____ Home Phone #_____

Family Physician: _____ Phone # _____

Last exam:_____

Parent or Guardian's Name:_____

Address:_____

City:_____Postal Code:_____ Home Phone # _____

Contact Person:_____ Phone #_____

Health Card #_____ Version ____

Who may we thank for referring ? _____

Cause of Disability (if known):_____

Level of Functioning: Self Help Skills : yes__ no__   Semi-Dependent: yes__ no__
                Totally Dependent: yes__ no__

Weight:_____Height: _____ Visually Impaired: yes__ no__ Hearing Impaired: yes__ no__

1. Please list any present medication names and daily dose:
    _____

2. Is patient allergic to OR reacted adversely to:
    a) any medicine   _____
    b) any foods   _____
     c) local anaesthesia_____
    d)latex products   _____
    e) other   _____
3. Has patient been hospitalised in the last 5 years? Yes __ no__. If yes, for what?
_____

4. Has patient had any serious trouble with any previous dental treatment, including
    abnormal bleeding? Yes__ No__?

5. Is patient on a special diet? _____ What kind?_____
6. Recent weight gain or loss? Yes__ No__
7. Does patient need assistance in feeding? Yes__ No__
8. Does patient gag or throw up easily? Yes__ No__
9. Who is responsible for brushing the patient's teeth? _____
   How often? _____
10. When was the patient's last dental treatment? _____
11. Does the patient exhibit any oral habits (finger sucking, hand biting, chew on objects, Grinding teeth, cloth habits, smoking, etc.)
12. Circle any of the following which the patient presently has or has had in the past:
    Seizures   Heart murmur   Cerebral Palsy   Congenital heart disease
    Hepatitis Artificial heart valve Liver disease   Heart surgery
    Kidney trouble   Shunt for fluid on brain   Jaundice
    Artificial joint   Diabetes   Asthma   High or low blood pressure
    Rheumatic fever Hay fever   Sores or growths in mouth   Thyroid disease
    Venereal disease   Tuberculosis Haemophilia or anaemia Persistent cough/nasal drainage
    Cortisone or steroid med.   AIDS/HIV   Stomach ulcers   Limited joint movement
    Heart trouble   Breathing difficulties   Pneumonia
13. Has the patient ever experienced any mental, sexual, or physical abuse?_____
14. Please add any other information you feel we should know concerning the patient's medical or dental health.
Date:_____ Signature:_____

Please review history and indicate any changes:
Relevant Changes:
date: _____

_____

signature _____

date: _____

_____

signature _____

date: _____

_____

signature _____

Oral Hygiene Skill Survey and Programme

Special Needs Dental Clinic Victoria Hospital

Patient Name: Hosp#:

Caregiver: Self Help Skills: Consult Date:

OBSERVATIONS OF TOOTHBRUSHING:

_____

SCORING KEY:

0 - step could not be completed	1 - caretaker completes step for individual
2 - need prompt to complete step	3 - step can be completed independently

STEPS DATES							
1. Identify own brush							
2. Approach sink							
3. Pick up and wet brush							
4. Put toothpaste on brush							
5. Put toothbrush in mouth							
6. Keep brush in mouth 5 secs							
7. Keep brush in mouth 1 min							
8. Keep brush in mouth 2 mins							
9. Brush inside/outside front teeth							
10. Brush inside/outside back teeth							
11. Brush chewing surfaces of teeth							
12. Rinse and spit							
13. Put toothbrush/toothpaste away							
PLAQUE INDEX							
BLEEDING INDEX							

PROGRAM RECOMMENDATIONS:

1. ◯ Monitor activity
2. ◯ No use of toothpaste
3. ◯ Fluoride rinse/Fluoride gel
4. ◯ Chlorhexidine rinse/brush/ swab
5. ◯ Re Dye Programme
6. ◯ Reinforcements
7. ◯ Verbal queuing

ADDITIONAL INSTRUCTION:

_____

_____

_____

_____

SUPPORT NEEDED:

Arm: _____

Head: _____

Hand over Hand: _____

Other: _____

_____

_____

FLOSS (please check one):

◯ Patient is able to floss
◯ Patient is able to floss with finger holder
◯ Patient is unable to floss; caregiver assistance needed
◯ Patient is unable to floss; no flossing technique currently used

CLASSIFICATION OF CLEANING SKILLS

◯ Patient requires significant assistance
◯ Patient has some dexterity but insufficient cleaning techniques
◯ Patient can effectively brush with little assistance
◯ Patient requires virtually no assistance

Reinforcers Used: (books, TV, food) _____

Toothbrush Adaptations Used: _____

Additional Comments and Goals: _____

fairly extensive mobile systems that allow for easy transportability and have thus enhanced the ability to provide care in remote area hospitals.

Selection of Patients to be treated in a hospital setting under general anaesthesia (see Chapters 6 and 7).

General Anaesthetic. Pre-operative instructions: In order to help prepare patients to better tolerate a procedure under general anaesthesia letters to the caregiver detailing expectations are often helpful. This letter may include such things as the admitting process, special services available, parking, accommodation, and if an in-patient, specifics about do's and don'ts prior to the procedure (*Form 3*). Some hospitals have special programmes where they allow pre-operative visits in an attempt to decrease anxiety[19]. With many of the more profoundly disabled individuals they help facilitate the process by decreasing the time spent in the hospital environment as much as possible. It is often a great help to the anaesthetist to have the primary care giver come with the patient to the operating room (O.R.) in order to assist in the provision of the general anaesthetic.

FORM 3

The Day of Surgery

IMPORTANT: Remember that (name) cannot have anything to eat or drink after midnight the day before surgery (unless otherwise instructed).

THINGS TO BRING TO THE HOSPITAL:
Your identification card
Your medical system payment card
Completed pre-op physical form.
Change of clothing as required
For anyone else: Something to read etc. while waiting during the surgery
Money for the parking lot.

Arrive at the Admitting Department of the Hospital at the time indicated in your confirmation letter. (Name) will receive their identification wrist bracelet and they will begin a chart. Staff there will direct you to the Day Surgery Unit.

Day Surgery Unit: (Name) will be examined by the nurses. If you have any concerns or questions it is important to let the nurses know at this time. (Name) will be assigned a hospital bed and given pyjama's to wear. Then (name) will be able to rest until they call from the operating room. The average length of stay here is about 3 hours.

During Surgery: The family waiting room is usually located just down the hall from the operating room. A nurse or volunteer will come to get you here after (name) surgery is complete and they are in the Recovery Room. This is a good time to get a bite to eat in the coffee bar.

Recovery Room: (Name) will be here anywhere from 5 minutes to ½ hour while they wake up from the anaesthesia. Only one person is allowed in this area. When (name) is awake the nurses will bring you and (name) to the post-op area.

Post Op: This is where you will stay until (name) is ready to go home. The nurses will monitor (name) and make sure that they have something to drink and go to the bathroom before discharging you. The length of stay here is dependent on (name); however, it is about 2 to 4 hours.

At home: Individuals tend to recover quickly. They may be very hungry and it is fine to give them small, light meals and lots of fluid. Quiet activity is recommended and you may find that they want to sleep. If you have any concerns, call your family doctor or the dental office.

Post-op Appointment: Someone should call on the Monday following (name) surgery to book a post-op appointment. This appointment is usually 6–8 weeks after surgery.

Pre –Admission Programme

What is a Pre-admission Clinic?
The Pre-Admission clinic is a 2–4 hour session to prepare you for your operation. At the clinic, you will be registered for your hospital admission and meet some of the staff who will explain how to prepare for your operation. You will spend time with a nurse, may see a medical specialist and/or an anaesthetist, and will have various tests done.

Is it necessary to attend the clinic?
Yes, if you do not attend, your operation may be cancelled.

How do I book my appointment at the Clinic?
Call Patient Registration, as directed by your doctor's office to arrange an appointment. Your Pre-Admission Clinic appointment should occur 14 to 28 days prior to surgery.

What if I cannot attend at the scheduled time?
It is necessary to reschedule your appointment, please notify Patient registration at least 72 hours (3 days) in advance. If you do not attend the clinic at your scheduled time, your procedure may be cancelled.

Do I need to bring anything with me on the day of my visit?
Yes, please bring:
any pills or medicine you are presently taking
your medical system payment card
completed documents that may have been given to you by your doctor
a family member/significant other is welcome to come to the clinic with you if you wish,
non-ambulatory patients requiring assistance must be accompanied
bring an interpreter with you if needed

Post Operative Management and Instructions

Upon completion of a procedure and transfer of the patient to the recovery room, the post-operative orders are written for patient care in the following areas. All orders prior to an O.R. procedure are no longer valid and must be rewritten. These would include the following as required.

- Vital signs
- Pain
- Swelling
- Haemorrhage
- Ventilation
- Medications
- Fluids and diet
- Ward care vs. ambulation
- Discharge information
- Post-operative follow up

For an example of how this may look see *addendum 4*.

General Anaesthetic. Hospital Post-Operative Note. A short note or summary of the procedures accomplished are written or dictated for the hospital record. Normally, dependent on the hospital the following are required:

- Patient name and hospital #
- Name of surgeon, anaesthetist, and assistant if any
- Pre Operative diagnosis
- Post Operative diagnosis
- Operation performed
- Clinical Note: In this note the following are normally detailed.
  - Age and gender of patient and reason they were admitted for a general anaesthetic procedure
  - Type of intubation and anaesthesia
  - Type dosage and effectiveness of pre-op medication
  - Radiographs taken
  - Description of procedure including draping, throat pack and use of rubber dam
  - Description of findings of exam and of sanative procedures used
  - List teeth restored and material used
  - List extractions, how done, and haemostasis accomplished. Detail amount of blood loss
  - Describe irrigation used and removal of throat pack
  - Describe how procedure tolerated and condition of patient on return to recovery room
  - Describe postoperative follow-up required[1]

Teaching and research

Introduction of competencies and proficiencies will assist in overall development of standards of care for populations with disabilities outside the institutions[4,20]. Funding programmes for interns vary considerably in different countries. In some hospitals in the United States the federal government funds the internships, whereas in Canada they are self funded by the work they do.

References

1. Zambito R F, Black H A, Tesch L B. *Hospital Dentistry Practice and Education*. St. Louis: Mosby, 1997.
2. Lockhart P B, Connoly S F, Sargent R K. *A Practical Guide to Hospital Dental Practice*. Ed 3. Portland, Oregon: JBK Publishing, 1991.
3. Waldman B, Swerdloff M, Perlman S. Children with disabilities: More than just numbers. *J Dent Child* 1999: **66:**192–196.
4. Van Ostenberg P. Navigating an educational program through the treacherous 90's: dynamics of the health care system. *J Dent Educ* 1991; **55:** 531–533.
5. Schoen M H, Marcus M, Koch A L. The hospital-sponsored dental services program. II an evaluation of dental services. *Spec Care Dent* 1988; **8:** 6–12
6. Schoen M H, Marcus M, Koch A L. An evaluation of the Robert Wood Johnson Foundation's Hospital Sponsored Ambulatory Dental Services Program. *Health Serv Res* 1987; **22:** 327–339.
7. Wehler-Randall C, White J D. Oral health status of Special Olympic Athletes. (submitted to IADR).
8. Fenton S J. 1993 survey of training in the treatment of persons with disabilities. *Interface* 1993; **971:** 3.
9. Romer M, Dougherty N, Amores-Lefleur E. Predoctoral education in special care dentistry: paving the way to better access? *J Dent Child* 1999; **66:** 132–135.
10. Gordon S M, Dionne R A et al. Dental fear and anxiety as a barrier to accessing oral health care among patients with special health care needs. *Spec Care Dent* 1998; **18:** 88–92.
11. Fenton S J. People with disabilities need more lip service (editorial). *Spec Care Dent* 1999; **19:** 198.
12. Perlman S, Friedman C, Tesini D. Prevention and Treatment Considerations for the dental patient with special needs. UARCO Professional Dental Care, _ HYPERLINK "mailto:J@J" __J@J_ consumer products Inc. Grandview Road, Skillman, NJ., Oct 1991.
13. Fetter C. *Specialised Care Company Oral Training Program* (workbook and video series) Hampton, NH.
14. Fetter C. *A Person Centred Approach to Handling Resistance to Daily Hygiene Services* (a workbook and video training series) Hampton, NH.
15. Tesini D, Dolan K M. *Oral Health Care for Community Residences: Improving Oral Health through Performance Measurement*. Tufts Dental Facilities
16. Glassman P, Miller C, Wozniak T, Jones C. A preventive dentistry training program for caretakers of persons with disabilities residing in community residential facilities. *Spec Care Dent* 1994; **14:** 137–143.
17. Narvey A. Personal communication. 1999.
18. *Guidelines for management of Paediatric Dental Patients Receiving Chemotherapy, Bone marrow Transplants, and or Radiation*. Academy of Paediatric Dentistry. Reference manual 1998–1999.
19. Kain Z N, Mayes L C, et al. Parental presence during induction of anaesthesia versus sedative premedication: which intervention is more effective? *Anesthesiology* 1998; **89:** 1147–1156
20. Chambers D W, Glassman P. A Primer on competency-based Evaluation. *J Dent Education* 1997; **61:** 651–666.

Cleft Palate Clinic – Treatment Protocol
(As used by Calgary Children's Hospital)

Age: Infant, 0–12 Months

DENTAL	Parent education 1) long term concerns; 2) early infant care; 3) feeding syndrome; 4) oral hygiene & fluoride
PLASTIC SURGERY	1) Maxillary Orthopaedics; 2) Study models, photos Cleft Lip repair Primary Cleft Lip
ORTHODONTICS	1) Neonatal orthopaedics
NURSING	1) Hospital visitation or contact with parents by telephone to provide support, information, handouts, feeding instructions and supplies with a goal towards normal weight gain
SOCIAL WORK	1) Seen by Clinic Social Worker either prior to or at time of paediatric evaluation.
PAEDIATRICS	Paediatric evaluation to assess infant's health and total well being at 4–6 weeks and again at 6 months, 12 months and 18 months to monitor growth and development.

Age: 10–14 weeks

NURSING	Lip repair pre- and post-operative teaching done.
SOCIAL WORK	Social Work intervention at time of lip and palatal surgery.
DENTAL	Weaning advice; fluoride reinforcement; teething advice

Age : 6–12 months

DENTAL	Initial dental examination 1) Nutrition; 2) Oral Hygiene instruction; 3) Prevention
NURSING	Minnesota Infant Development Inventory (MIDI) reviewed with team and assessments scheduled accordingly. Involved in pre and post-operative teaching in preparation for palatal surgery
SPEECH	Parents receive: MIDI at 6 months or Minnesota Communicative Development Inventory (MCDI) at 12 months. If the above parent questionnaire reveals difficulties, bringing for assessment of a) cognition b) oral facial exam c) voice d) preverbal development skills and provide the appropriate intervention from results of the assessment.
AUDIOLOGY	Initial hearing test at 6–8 months. If results normal, review in 6 months, 1 year and then upon request. If abnormal findings, hearing test should be repeated every 3 months until normal. Copy of audiogram to family physician.

Age: Toddler, 12–18 months

DENTAL	Dental preventive programme. Nutritional counselling important.

PLASTIC SURGERY	Cleft palate repair in some centres
RECORDS	Study models, photos
NURSING	Involved in pre- and post-operative teaching in preparation for palatal surgery in some centres. Arrange for ENT referral for tube insertions if necessary. MCDI sent to parents.
SPEECH	If the MCDI or MIDI come back as normal, there will be no assessment until after palate repair for cleft lip children around age 2.

Age: Preschool, 2–5 years

DENTAL	Speech appliances if indicated Orthodontics – ideally should be linked to timing for surgical procedures, i.e. lip and nose revision, grafting if indicated. Establish orthodontics/pedodontics/plastics long term treatment plan.
ORTHODONTICS	Space maintenance
RECORDS	Study models, photos; Panorex, periapicals
SPEECH	Assess all children between ages of 2 and 5 for: a) oral facial exam; b) voice evaluation; c) articulation test; d) language test – receptive & expressive; e) fluency screen. Difficulties in any of the above areas will result in appropriate treatment intervention.
AUDIOLOGY	Able to do headphone testing.
SOCIAL WORK	Contact with parents at beginning of formal speech and socialisation.

Age: School age, 6–9 years

DENTAL	Need for cleaning pre-surgery. Preliminary alignment. Combined Paedodontic/Orthodontic/Surgical intervention. Aesthetics becomes a consideration when child identifies it is a problem.
PLASTIC SURGERY	Lip/nasal revision; Pharyngoplasty; Columella lenghtening Secondary alveolar bone graft (lip, nasal revision); Pharyngoplasty
ORAL SURGERY	Secondary alveolar bone graft; Ectopic eruptions; Supernumeraries
ORTHODONTICS	Crossbite correction; Arch expansion; Anterior dental alignment; preliminary retention.
RECORDS	Comprehensive orthodontic records. Study models, photos; Panorex, ceph (lateral antero/posterior) TMJ as required
NURSING	Participate in pre- and post- op teaching for secondary surgical procedures.
SPEECH	All new patients of school age will be assessed in the following areas: a) oral facial exam; b) voice evaluation – nasoendoscopy as necessary; c) articulation test; d) language skills will be screened

Age: Pre-Adolescent, 10–13 years

DENTAL	Routine care. Cosmetic dentistry when identified as a problem. Graft evaluation for purpose of potential implants. CT or MRI scan (Expan-

sion must be complete). Not recommended if orthognathic surgery considered

ORTHODONTICS   Comprehensive orthodontic treatment including records

NURSING   Determine individual need for follow-up and schedule accordingly

SOCIAL WORK   Social work intervention throughout adolescence

Age: Late Adolescent, 13–18 years

PLASTIC SURGERY Final revisions; Septo-rhinoplasty

ORTHODONTICS   Comprehensive orthodontic treatment including records

NURSING   Be available to field questions. Provide information and counselling, as necessary

SPEECH   Will assess voice and articulation and refer as appropriate

Age: Adult, 18+

DENTAL   Adult prosthetic considerations linked to periodontal status

ORAL SURGERY   Orthognathic surgery; Third molar extractions

ORTHODONTICS   Comprehensive orthodontic treatment; TMJ as required

Protocol for Cardiac Patients

- The primary objectives for this protocol would be :
- Decrease the morbidity and mortality due to infection.
- Decrease the morbidity due to haemorrhage
- Facilititate the patient's nutritional status
- Improve the patient's comfort
- Increase the education of the patient,family, and physician relative to the importance of maintaining oral health and the methods to achieve it.

Antibiotic Prophylaxis Recommendation for Oral Procedures

Situation	Agent	Protocol*
Standard General Prophylaxis	Amoxicillin	Adults: 2.0g Children: 50 mg/kg orally 1 hour before procedure
Unable to take oral medications	Ampicillin	Adults: 2.0g. intra-muscularly (IM) or intravenously (IV) Children: 50 mg/kg IM or IV within 30 minutes before procedure
Allergic to penicillin	Clindamycin OR Cephalexin** or Cefadroxil** OR Azithromycin or Clarithromycin	Adults: 500 mg Children: 20 mg/kg orally 1 hour before procedure Adults: 2.0g Children: 50 mg/kg orally 1 hour before procedure Adults: 500 mg Children: 15 mg/kg orally 1 hour before procedure
Allergic to penicillin and unable to take oral medications	Clindamycin OR Cefazolin**	Adults: 800 mg Children: 20 mg/kg IV within 30 Adults: 1.0 g Children: 25 mg/kg IM or IV within 30 minutes before procedure

*Total children's dose should not exceed adult dose
**Cephaloeporine should not be used in individuals with immediate-type hypersensitivity reaction furticaria, angiodema, or anaphylaxis to penicillins

Patients at potential increased risk of hematogenous total joint infection[1]

Immunocompromised/Immunosuppressed patients

- Inflammatory arthropathies; rheumatoid arthritis, systemic lupus erythamatosus
- Disease, drug or radiation-induced immunosuppression

Other patients

- Insulin-dependent (Type 1) diabetes
- First two years following joint placement
- Previous prosthetic joint infections
- Malnourishment
- Haemophilia

[1]Advisory Statement. Antibiotic Prophylaxis for Dental Patient with Total Joint Replacement. *JADA* 1997; **126:**1008.

Protocol for Bone Marrow Transplant (BMT)

PATIENTS

BMT PRE-OP CONSIDERATIONS:

General Health Concerns:

Medical History

>Document type and stage of cancer, current medications, allergies and any relevant past medical conditions

Transplant Information

>Document the type of BMT transplant (autogenic, allogenic, umbilical cord)

Venous Catheter Protection

>Prescribe prophylactic antibiotics prior to treatment (Drug dosing: follow AHA Guidelines)

Oral Health Concerns:

Soft and Hard Tissue

Gingival and Periodontal health:

>Document baseline periodontal condition, assessing gingival health and alveolar bone loss
>
>Identify periodontal pathogens via crevicular fluid cultures as needed
>
>Perform oral prophylaxis to remove plaque and calculus

Exfoliation concerns:

>Remove mobile primary teeth (or those expected to exfoliate within 3 months of BMT)

Eruption concerns:

>Evaluate ectopically erupting teeth for pathology or potential bacterial reservoir
>
>Evaluate partially-erupted permanent teeth (6y, 12y, 3rd molars) for increased risk of pericoronitis

Caries:

>Prevent caries by sealant and fluoride application
>
>Restore carious lesions and do pulp therapy as indicated
>
>Remove teeth with periapical or furcal pathology

Growth and Development

Orthodontic appliances:

>Remove appliances that contribute to poor oral hygiene or mucosal irritation

Post Operative Orders

The following orders would be written on the patients hospital chart prior to leaving the operating room.

Post-operative orders

Check vital signs q15 min. until stable.

Suction prn. for haem. – replace gauze packs prn. for haem.

Ice packs to surgical areas – 20 min on 20 min off

Continue I.V. at   rate   or discontinue if no longer tolerated.

Medication as required - Detail

Pain

Antibiotic

Nausea and vomiting

Normal medications

Encourage clear liquid

Discharge to Guardian when stable

Post Operative appointment at   #   in   weeks.

Call #   if problems arise.

Chapter 14

Domiciliary Dental Care

Janice Fiske and Debbie Lewis

Definition

Domiciliary dental care (DDC) is: "a service that reaches out to care for those people who cannot reach a service themselves"[1]. It includes dental care carried out in an environment where a person is resident either permanently or temporarily, as opposed to care delivered in dental clinics or mobile units. The aim of DDC is to deliver appropriate oral health care to people whose circumstances make it impossible, unreasonable or otherwise impractical for them to secure care in a fixed clinic, hospital or dental mobile unit[2].

Increasing demand

The demand for DDC is increasing and is likely to continue to do so[3]. The reasons for this increasing demand include:

a) A growing disabled population

Improvements in sanitation, infant survival and medical science have contributed to increased life expectancy in industrialised and urbanised countries (*Figure 1*). Consequently, more people are surviving with illness and disability, and many of them are reaching old age. According to Bennett and Morreale[4], in 1996, 70% of Canadians over the age of 65 years remained functionally independent. Whilst a large proportion of elderly people fall into this category, the majority of all disabled people are elderly. In the UK there are 6.5 million disabled people, equivalent to one in eight of the population, of whom 60% are over the

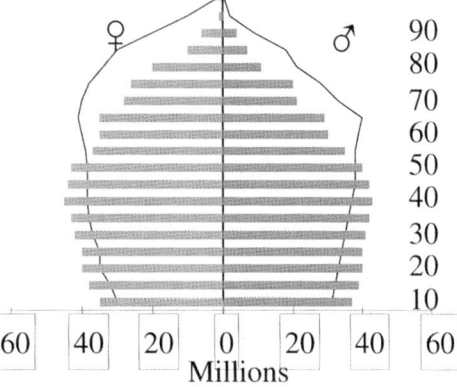

Figure 1

Population projections for the developed world, the solid bars represent the size of their respective age cohorts in 1998, the line is the outline of the structure in 2050 (Source: United Nations 1998 revision of world population estimates and projections).

143

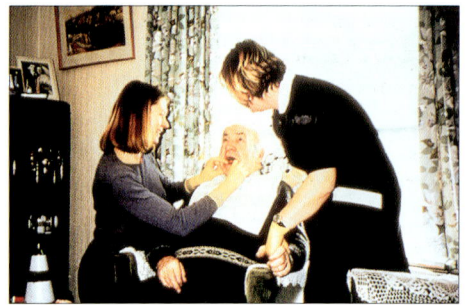

Figure 2

Dental care being provided for a resident in a home for elderly people (Reprinted by kind permission of the Editor, Dental Update)

age of 65[5]. Twenty percent of people over the age of 85 years are either house-bound or bed-bound.

In Northern Europe it is estimated that 4–7 % of the population live in long-stay residential care. Whilst there are no official statistics for the proportion of elderly people that are bed-ridden or house-bound, it is estimated that 12–14 % of the elderly population fall into this category. This proportion represents significant numbers of elderly people – approximately one and a half million in the UK and approximately seven million in the USA. Thus, there are increasing numbers of frail and medically compromised elderly people. Their mobility and/or ability for self-care is often reduced by physical disability, mental impairment or disease. A combination of functional limitation, multiple drug use and limited access to dental care puts them at greater risk of poor oral health.[6,7] The oral health of residents in nursing homes and long-term care facilities has been reported as poor in many European countries[8–13]. These reports have revealed the need for dental care both within long-stay accommodation and for housebound elderly people living in private homes or sheltered accommodation[14–16] (*Figure 2*). It may be unreasonable or impractical for people who are house-bound and living in institutions to attend a dental surgery for treatment. Their oral health needs will remain unmet unless they are able to access domiciliary dental care services (DDCS).

b) Legislation

Increasing awareness about equal opportunities for people with disabilities has led to legislation in many countries. For example, *The Disability Discrimination Act 1995 (DDA)* in the UK has implications for dentists and the provision of domiciliary dental care as it makes the removal of barriers to disabled people's participation in society a legal requirement[17]. From October 1999, the DDA required service providers to act fairly and to be flexible by taking action to remove any barriers excluding disabled people. The Act defines discrimination in two ways. Firstly, it defines it as "failure to provide a reasonable adjustment". As far as dentists are concerned, where dental premises create a physical barrier to access, the dentist has to consider providing the service by a "reasonable alternative means". For example, if a dental surgery is up a flight of stairs and inaccessible to a disabled person, it requires the dentist to offer domiciliary care. The second definition relates to "less favourable treatment" which is unlawful for a reason related to disability (where it can not be justified under the terms of the Act) even where a provider treats a person less favourably or refuses to serve them because they think this is for the disabled person's own good. For example, because they think that the person is incapable of benefiting from the service or that another agency would provide a service which would suit the disabled person's needs better. Not only does the Act open the door to an increased demand for DDCS, it also opens the door to possible litigation if such a service is not offered.

In the USA, *The Americans with Disabilities Act 1990* requires that all health care providers make reasonable accommodations to facilitate access to care[18]. Additionally, the State boards of dentistry, which govern the practice of dentistry, must ensure that every dental practice maintains the community standard of care. Thus, the ethical, legal and regulatory mandates for equal access and equal standards are very clear[19].

c) Increasing public awareness

DDCS are still not widely known about. Even when they are, there remains a public perception that only oral examinations and simple dental procedures can be carried out in the domiciliary setting[6]. Despite this perception, a recent study looking at barriers to dental care in frail and functionally dependent older adults reports that the majority of them expressed a preference for treatment to be carried out in their own homes[20]. Knowledge about the DDA, dental advertising, and word of mouth about DDCS from friends and relatives will lead to greater demand for domiciliary care.

d) An increasingly dentate disabled population

Studies from many industrialised countries indicate that changes are occurring in the dental demographic picture for elderly people and that more people are surviving into old age with at least some of their natural teeth. Data from the 1998 Adult Dental Health Survey in the UK show that among UK adults aged 75 years and over, 42% had retained some of their teeth and 10% had more than 20 teeth[21]. It appears that the older age groups are keeping more of their teeth, are more likely to have had teeth restored, and have a larger number of artificial crowns than in previous decades[21]. As dentate elderly people become disabled they are more likely to use dental services regularly than edentate elderly people do. This will not only increase the demand for DDCS, it will also require the skills and equipment to provide a more comprehensive service than those required for the provision of complete dentures[22]. The oft reported high normative need for dental care (commonly exceeding 70%) has demonstrated the growing requirement for both preventive strategies and complex restorative procedures amongst this sector of the population.

In summary, an increasing demand for domiciliary care is based on:

- a growing population of disabled people
- legislative pressure
- increasing public awareness – 'advocacy'
- an increasingly dentate population

Domiciliary visiting patterns

Most dentists provide little DDC. In the UK, on average, a National Health Service dentist provides home care for 2.9 patients per month[3,23]. The majority of visits are made out of regular office hours, either on the dentist's way into work or way home[23]. Routine services are typically inexpensive, short duration procedures which have successful outcomes in the majority of cases, with treatment provision mainly limited to examinations, hygiene procedures, denture provision and simple extractions[3,4,19,23]. This is probably realistic, although, the advent of adhesive filling materials and techniques, for example, atraumatic restorative technique (ART), allows restorations and adhesive bridges to be added to this treatment list.

Dentists not providing DDCS state their reasons as:

- not feeling adequately prepared or up to date in this area[4]
- insufficient demand for the service
- poor remuneration
- inadequate equipment
- reduced quality of work[24]

Dental Care Delivery Systems

Whilst it is usually more convenient and cost effective to treat patients in the surgery, for some people the physical, emotional or psychological trauma of being transported to a dental surgery and the reliance on the availability of a carer may negate any benefits provided by the surgery environment. Therefore, it is preferable to provide treatment on-site, at home, for some client groups despite the inconvenience that this may cause the dental team[19]. This may take the form of:

a) Permanent fixed clinics in residential homes

Whilst providing access to a comprehensive dental service, they are too expensive to build, maintain and staff in all but the very largest facilities.

b) Mobile units

Shaver[25] and Combs[26] described two types of mobile units. The first is a fully equipped dental vehicle which is essentially a 'walk-in' dental surgery and delivers a service inside the van. However, it requires patients to be transported outside the home and needs a tail-lift to facilitate wheelchair access (see Chapter 1, figure 2). The second is an equipment van delivering a complete dental office that can be set up on-site in an individual's home. The advantages of these services are that they provide easy access to a conventional dental setting which can supply all types of dental services. The main disadvantage is the cost of setting up the service. Both the equipment van and the dental vehicle are more likely to visit institutions or day-centres for elderly people than housebound individuals, as this minimises difficulties with travelling, parking, setting-up and accessing power sources whilst maximising the numbers of patients treated in a defined time period.

Figure 3

Domiciliary equipment being used at the bedside of a patient in a nursing home (Reprinted by kind permission of the Editor, Dental Update)

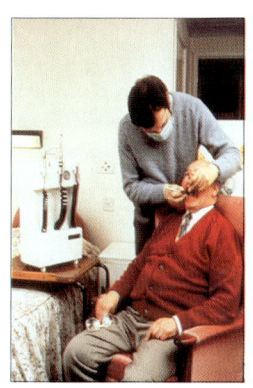

c) Portable dental equipment or domiciliary dental care

This is the most effective alternative and the only system able to provide dental care for people who are confined to bed or a chair (*Figure 3*).

d) A 'mix and match' approach

This mixes domiciliary and surgery-based care and matches it to the complexity of the dental procedures. It can be adopted for some people. For example, anxious patients may feel able to attend the surgery once establishing a rapport with the dental team on a domiciliary basis has helped to reduce their fear. Regular review of an individual's need for DDCS is advocated as improved health may mean that some people are able to return to attending the dental surgery. Furthermore, experience shows that people are generally prepared to make the effort required to visit the surgery in the knowledge that it is only necessary occasionally. Thus, it may be prudent to use a minimum number of well-planned visits to the dental surgery to perform technical or complex procedures (such as a surgical extraction for a person on anticoagulation therapy) whilst carrying out other procedures in the home (such as denture provision).

Client Groups

Domiciliary care normally involves visiting :

- residential units and nursing homes
- day hospitals
- day centres
- individuals' own homes

but it can also encompass visiting people:

- in hospitals
- palliative care units
- hostels for homeless people.

The majority of people requiring domiciliary care are elderly but a significant number of younger disabled people can also benefit from care at home. The client groups most likely to require DDCS are people with: physical disabilities causing problems with mobility; medical conditions leading to disability – such as chronic obstructive airway disease, emphysema, stroke, Parkinson's disease, etc.; conditions where people become disorientated, confused or panicked when removed from a familiar environment – such as autism, Alzheimer's disease and agoraphobia; learning or mental disability that causes difficulty in making and keeping surgery-based appointments; and severe dental anxiety and phobia such that people feel unable to enter a dental surgery.

The Domiciliary Dental Team

Members of the team will vary from country to country depending on the legislation controlling the delivery of health care, but will normally include the dentist, dental nurse and dental hygienist.

Advantages and disadvantages of domiciliary dental care

These have been described by Christensen and Fiske[27] as:

Advantages of DDC for the dental team

- An opportunity to learn more about the client in their own surroundings and, thus, to provide a holistic approach to care. It gives access to medication and any patient- kept medical notes, as well as providing clues about eating habits. It allows an assessment of the person's ability to comply with oral hygiene advice, for example can the individual get to a bathroom/sink, stand/sit at the sink and manage tooth-brushing.
- The client is usually more comfortable and relaxed in the surroundings of their own environment, rapport is improved and there may be more compliance with treatment and preventive regimes.

- The patient seems to be more interested in their treatment, thus motivation and compliance may be increased
- Increased access to carers
- A change of environment
- Valued and appreciated more
- A reduction in the frustrations of failed appointments and waiting for transport to arrive

Advantages of DDC for the client/patient
- Increased access to care
- Increased independence from reliance on someone else to take them to the dentist
- The opportunity to be treated in their own environment
- Decreased fear of the unknown
- Increased control/power over events
- Increased ability or inclination to disclose personal information, or to ask questions, as confidentiality is increased.
- A feeling of importance
- Having a visitor/guest
- Peer group support in residential settings

Disadvantages of DDC for the dental team
- Being out of their own environment of the conventional dental setting which often leads to a feeling of a lack of control
- Increased fear of the unknown
- Decreased control/power
- Lack of emergency back-up
- Lack of hygiene control
- Making compromises, such as posture, lighting and lack of radiographic facilities
- More difficult not to become involved with a client's personal life and problems
- Decreased time for patient care because of increased time spent travelling
- Increased stress
- Increased vulnerability to personal safety

Disadvantages of DDC for the client/patient
- DDCS are not widely known about
- Limited scope of dental procedures available
- Limited choice of dentist
- Difficult to miss appointments
- Uncertainty of strangers visiting
- Invasion of privacy
- Disruption of routine for both the client and their carer
- Embarrassment regarding physical/social circumstances

Knowledge and Skills

Domiciliary care requires the dental team to transfer its skills from the dental surgery to the kitchen, sitting room or the bedroom whilst respecting the individual's culture, wishes and home[27]. The domiciliary dental team can benefit from developing a knowledge and understanding of conditions leading to impairments and disabilities and how they can effect oral health. A good knowledge of medical conditions and their associated problems, gerodontics, the causes and management of medical emergencies and the use of domiciliary equipment is important. Teamwork is fundamental to the organisation and smooth running of DDCS; whilst, flexibility, improvisation, anticipation and assertiveness are necessary to meet the plethora of differing environments and circumstances encountered.

In summary, the knowledge and skills required are:
- conditions leading to impairment
- use of domiciliary equipment
- gerodontics
- ability to be flexible, innovative
- networking
- communication skills
- management of medical emergencies
- team working

Training issues

Not surprisingly research has established that dentists are more likely to provide DDCS if they have already provided such care or if they have been shown how to do it[1,28,29]. Until recently, training in dentistry in the undergraduate curriculum (even within geriatric dentistry) has, on the whole, been confined to ambulatory people attending dental hospitals[29]. Thus, experience in DDCS was not gained until individuals were required to provide this modality of care. Fortunately, this picture is changing[28]. However, when staff who do not have DDCS experience join a practice, they require training in order to develop and maintain the knowledge and skills necessary for providing domiciliary care. This may be provided by accompanying an already experienced clinician.

Additionally, it is prudent for them to be trained in basic life support in order to deal with emergency situations which may arise in the home; manual handling to avoid personal injury whilst lifting and carrying domiciliary equipment; and health and safety issues to promote safe practice.

In summary, additional training that is required centres around:
- 'shadowing' an experienced clinician

- regular updating in basic life support
- knowledge of manual handling skills
- familiarity with health and safety legislation

Cost and Remuneration

The provision of oral care to disabled people is more time consuming than the provision of oral care to non-disabled people. This means that their care comes at a higher cost. This cost is even greater when the care is provided outside the conventional dental setting, whether it is via mobile dental units or domiciliary dental care. Whilst the occasional example exists of a dentist setting up a mobile dental service or dedicating a practice to domiciliary dental care, this is the exception rather than the rule[25,26]. Additionally, such services tend to be targeted at elderly people in residential care where reasonable numbers of patients can be seen per visit. Scientific and clinical evidence strongly support the health benefits, minimal risks and cost effectiveness of providing oral health care services to the long-term care population[19]. However, the provision of dental care for individual house-bound people is not viewed as an attractive financial proposition. Indeed, it is often not a viable financial proposition.

Dentists can not be expected to deliver more than the occasional home-based dental visit if there is no financial incentive to do so. This begs the question who should pay for the service – the Government, the Local Authority, or the disabled individual? This will vary according to the system of payment for health care within a country. Unless these issues are resolved, disabled people living in non-residential settings are at risk of being denied access to continuing oral care services.

Domiciliary equipment

The equipment and materials required by a practice depend on the number and type of visits planned and the resources available to purchase them. The principle to remember in assembling a domiciliary kit is: KISS – Keep It So Simple! Unless planning to do a reasonable number of home visits on a regular basis, most practices will find it adequate to have a basic examination kit, a prosthetic kit (including a portable handpiece), a small box of hand instruments and an adhesive filling material, and a selection of extraction forceps. A convenient method of housing the examination and prosthetic units is a "baby-care" box. A small compartmentalised tool-box can be used for hand instruments and filling materials. Provided the kits are restocked after each visit, they are ready for anyone in the practice to pick up and use.

DDC restricted mainly to the provision of dentures and simple extractions places little demand on the provision of domiciliary equipment.

The most sophisticated item required is a motor with a straight hand-piece for denture adjustments. A rechargeable, battery-operated motor requires a relatively small financial investment which can have a high return in terms of usefulness and convenience. They can be purchased with straight hand-pieces only or with both straight and contra-angled hand-pieces.

The increasing demand for DDCS by dentate people has led to the development of portable, restorative dental units. Purchase of a portable dental unit is a considerable financial investment. It requires research to find out which of the available units best fits your needs. Ideally, arrange a 'road test' before buying the unit. Units which house a compressor range in weight from approximately 7–17 kgms. Units without compressors are much lighter, but require either a separate compressor or compressed gas cylinders to run them (*Figure 4a–c*).

Lighting can range in sophistication. An angle-poise lamp with a clamp for use on a chair-back or table edge is useful. A portable fibre-optic light can help to diagnose caries in the absence of radiographic facilities[27]. Portable dental chairs are available, but they add extra weight and bulk to the domiciliary kit. Christensen and Fiske[27] point out that some elderly and disabled people feel particularly vulnerable when receiving dental care in the reclined position, and, in situations where the dentist can work from in front of the patient, an upright chair with a cushion for a head support against a wall may be suitable. However, the lack of a dental chair can jeopardise the operator's posture. From an ergonomic point of view, the dentist may prefer to stand behind the seated patient whilst supporting the patient's head against the dentist's body. When taking lower impressions or scaling lower teeth, kneeling in front of the patient puts the dentist at a height where good posture and comfort can be maintained. *Tables 1 and 2* list some items of available domiciliary equipment and a domiciliary kit checklist.

Treatment planning

Time management and planning

A dedicated time during the week for the provision of domiciliary care is more cost-effective than responding to the need on an ad hoc basis. Similarly having a basic dedicated domiciliary kit (which can be added to as required) is time saving. Obviously, there will be occasional, emergency domiciliary visits to be made outside the 'dedicated' time. However, forward planning helps to prevent problems and maximise the use of available time and resources. In the authors' experience, it is useful, prior to the first visit, to: telephone to clarify the dental problem and the need for a domiciliary visit; check the full and correct address and any helpful directions; enquire about parking facilities;

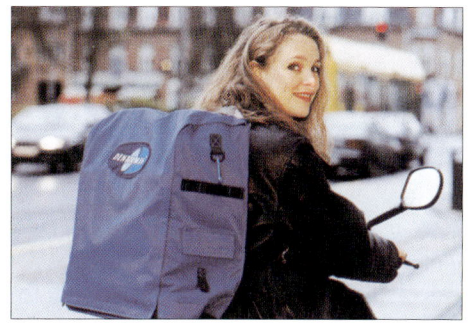

Figure 4a

The DentalMan™ unit is lightweight and portable

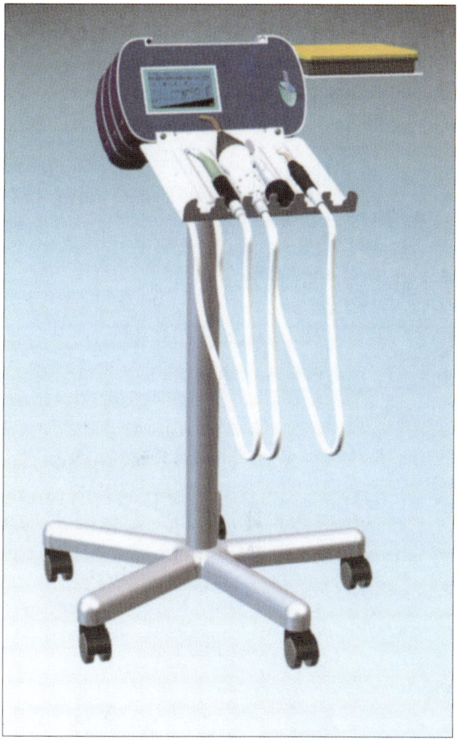

Figure 4b

The DentalMan™ unit set up for surgery use

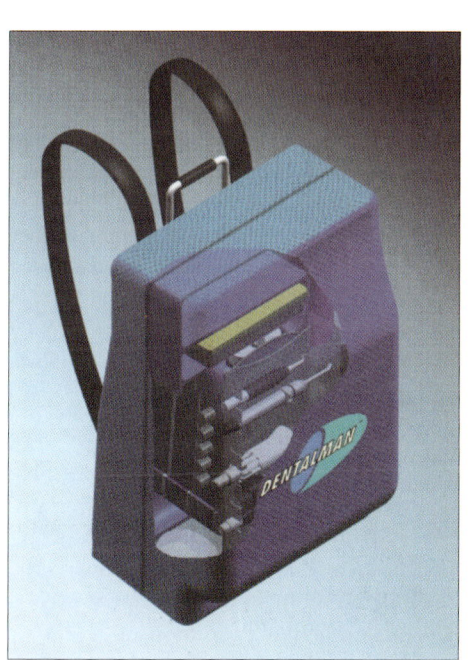

Figure 4c

Close-up of the DentalMan™ kit including the integral compressor

Table I. Domiciliary equipment details

Name	Manufacturer	Approximate price (excluding VAT)
Portable units		
Eddystone Gocase	Eddystone dental company	£2,800
Mini-dent domiciliary unit	Dentronic	£5,800
Pac-1	A-Dec Dental	£2,500
Portable dental surgical unit	Den-doc	£5,850
Dentalman™ Compact	Dentalman International A/S	£10,000
Portable handpieces (rechargeable)		
Etelna micromotor	Orthomax	£410
Derota	Quayle	£300
Dentalman™ Cordless instruments (handpieces, mirror light and lightcure)	Dentalman International A/S	£900
Light source		
Lightpen	Quayle	£275
Voroscope MXL	Garth Jessamine Healthcare	£175
Portable headrest	Ambulance Safety Systems, Yeovil	£85
Heat source		
Safe Air	Healthco	£85
Carrying boxes		
Baby box	Mothercare	£18

send a medical history questionnaire for completion and return; determine any special requirements, such as the need for the presence of a carer or a translator, collection of a key from a neighbour, etc.; and send a written appointment confirming the visit. These are tasks which can be delegated to the practice manager or receptionist.

The same principles are applied in the domiciliary environment as in the dental surgery setting, with the emphasis on prevention. In many instances there will be a need to discuss the management of patients with complex medical conditions with their general medical practitioner or hospital consultant prior to drawing up a definitive management regimen. In a situation where domiciliary care is required over a short period of time only (for example, a person recovering from a fractured neck of femur) it is reasonable to delay the provision of elective dental procedures until they can visit the surgery.

The provisional treatment plan, the need for further investigations, the possibility of any changes to the treatment plan and the timetable for treatment needs are discussed with the patient and /or carer and recorded in the patient notes. In the case of people with learning disabilities or mental illness, consideration must also be given to the issue of informed consent (See chapter 3). In such a situation, it is good practice to gain a second health-professional opinion (a doctor or

Table 2. Domiciliary kit suggestions

The equipment required will depend on the number and type of visits planned and the resources available to purchase it. However, the following checklist may be helpful.

General	Portable light	Portable suction
	Infection control items and equipment:	
	Gloves	*Masks/Face visors*
	Protective clothing for dentist and nurse, e.g. plastic aprons	
	Sharps disposal	*Disinfection solution*
	Liquid soap	*Plastic over-sheaths/cling film*
	Waste bags	*Paper towels, rolls, tissues*
	Dirty instrument-carrying receptacle	*Protective spectacles for patient*
	Laerdal resuscitation pocket mask	Emergency drugs kit / oxygen
Administrative	Identification badge	Prescription pad
	Diary	BNF
	Appointment cards	Mobile phone
	Record cards	Pen
	Referral forms	A - Z Route Map
	Laboratory forms	Change for parking
	Post-op instruction leaflets	Medical history forms
	Health promotion literature	Consent forms
Prosthetic Kit	Impression material	Scalpel
	Impression trays and mixing equipment	Shade guide
	Safe air heater	Articulation paper
	Portable motor, handpieces and burs	Plastic bags
	Waxes	Gauze
	Pressure relief paste	Cotton wool rolls
	Bite registration material	Vaseline
	Wax knife	Denture fixative
	Bite gauge	Dividers
	Paint scraper/ occlusal rim trimmer	Indelible pencil
Conservation kit	Portable unit (motor and suction)	
	Handpieces and burs	
	Light source	
	Syringes, needles, needleguards	
	Mirrors	
	Conservation instruments and tray	
Materials	Temporary dressing materials	Dry socket medicament
	Filling materials	Local anaesthetic cartridges
	Matrix bands	Topical anaesthetic cream/spray
	Gauze	Suture materials
	Cotton rolls and pellets	Haemostatic agents
	Vaseline	Bite packs
Periodontal kit	Hand scalers	Portable ultrasonic scaler
	Toothbrushes/pastes/therapeutic agents, e.g. Corsodyl, Omnigel	
Surgical kit	Forceps	Elevators
	MOS instruments including instuments for suturing	

(This list is an *aide memoire,* and is not prescriptive. Other items may be included according to individual preference).

another dentist) that the proposed treatment is in the best interests of the patient. In some countries it is a medico-legal requirement to do so. Also, it is prudent to involve a family member or carer even though this may have no legal standing in some countries (for example, in the UK where no-one can give consent on behalf of another adult). In this way an appropriate and realistic treatment plan can be negotiated and agreed before the individual is issued with a written treatment plan and estimation of cost (where charges are incurred).

Health and Safety

Domiciliary care involves a wide variety of environments and the dental team may not always have complete control over the conditions in which they find themselves working. However, privacy, confidentiality, access to water and electricity, and adequate lighting must always be ensured. There are a number of health and safety issues which must be addressed.

Risk assessment of the environment becomes routine at each new establishment. For example, ensuring that there is an obstacle-free passage from the patient to the work surface, water source, etc.; routinely using a circuit-breaker plug on all electrical appliances; and employing safe practice such as avoiding the use of naked flames.

Infection control in the domiciliary setting utilises the same principles which are applied in the dental surgery. All environments can be zoned for identification of clean and dirty areas, and disposable items used whenever possible. Dirty instruments must be kept separate from the domiciliary kit and transported in rigid containers and sharps must be transported in a sealed sharps container. Any local guidelines for disposal of clinical waste in the home should be complied with. In their absence, it is reasonable to dispose of non-sharp waste in the household rubbish as this is what would happen if the person had a nose bleed. If working in an establishment, such as a residential home, where bags for disposal of clinical waste and sharps containers are available, they can be utilised. Any waste which is to be transported back to the surgery should be double bagged and transported in a rigid container[30].

Safety of the individual and their home is paramount. People should be dissuaded from allowing strangers access to their home without proper identification and the dental team should encourage good practice by carrying and showing identification.

By virtue of the nature of the patients being treated there is greater chance of encountering a medical emergency on a domiciliary visit than in the dental surgery. Thus, due consideration must be given to both carrying, and the ability to use, oxygen and emergency drugs. As a minimum the dentist should carry a Laerdal mask to facilitate cardiopulmonary resuscitation should it be necessary and a mobile phone so that the emergency services can be called. If oxygen is carried, not only, must health and safety guidelines on transportation of flammable gases be complied with, but also, the vehicle's insurance company should be informed.

Personal safety is also important. It is prudent to have a third party present when a dentist, dental hygienist or other team member makes a home visit. It is recommended that the dentist/hygienist should be accompanied by another member of the dental team in an individual's home, and accompanied by a staff member or a member of the dental team in a residential home or hospital. Personal alarms and/or mobile telephones should be carried by the dental team. In accordance with manual handling training and guidelines, domiciliary equipment and materials should be transported on a trolley when possible; and patients should only be lifted or moved using proper procedures.

References

1. Fiske J. Over the threshold: Domiciliary dental care. *Talking Points for Dental Hygienists* 1992; **8:** 4–5.
2. All Wales Special Interest Group in Special Clinical Needs. *Guidelines for the Delivery of a Domiciliary Dental Service.* 1997.
3. Burke F J T, McCord J F, Hoad-Reddick G, Cheung S W. Provision of domiciliary care in a UK urban area: results of a survey. *Primary Dent Care* 1995; **2:** 47–50.
4. Bennett S, Morreale J. Providing care for elderly patients. *Ontario Dent* 1996; **73:** 44–54.
5. Martin J, White A, Meltzer H. *OPCS surveys of disability in Great Britain. Report 4. Disabled adults: services, transport and employment.* 1989. HMSO: London.
6. Fiske J, Gelbier S, Watson R M. Barriers to Dental Care in an elderly population resident in an inner city area. *J Dent* 1990; **18:** 236–242.
7. Strayer M S, Ibrahim M F. Dental treatment needs of homebound and nursing home patients. *Community Dent Oral Epidemiol* 1991; **19:** 176–177.
8. Manderson R D, Ettinger R L. Dental status of the institutionalised elderly population of Edinburgh. *Community Dent Oral Epidemiol* 1975; **3:** 100–107.
9. Smith J, Sheiham A. Dental treatment needs and demands of an elderly population in England. *Community Dent Oral Epidemiol* 1980; **8:** 360–364.
10. Hoad-Reddick G, Grant A A. The dental health of an elderly population in North-West England: Results of a survey undertaken in the Halton Health Authority. *J Dent* 1987; **15:** 138–146.
11. Nordenram G, Bohlin E. Dental status in the elderly a review of the Swedish literature. *Senior Citizen's Welfare Prog* 1981; **9:** 1–66.
12. Makila E. Oral health among the inmates of old people's homes III: Dentures and prosthetic aspects. *Proc Finn Dent Soc* 1977; **73:** 99–116.
13. Vigild M. denture status and need for prosthetic treatment among institutionalised elderly in Denmark. *Community Dent Oral Epidemiol* 1987; **15:** 128–133.
14. Hogan J I. A domiciliary dental service to the housebound from an Inner London health centre. *Community Dent Oral Epidemiol* 1986; **3:** 117–127.
15. Tobias T, Smith J M. Barriers to dental care and associated oral status and treatment needs in an elderly population living in sheltered accomodation in West Essex. *Br Dent J* 1987; **163:** 293–295.
16. MacEntee M I, Weiss R, Waxler-Morrison N E, Morrison B J. Factors influencing oral health in long term care facilities. *Community Dent Oral Epidemiol* 1987; **15:** 314–316.
17. *Disability Discrimination Act 1995.* Book no: 0105450952 (HMSO Publication) Now the Stationery Office.
18. *The Americans with Disabilities Act.* P.L. 101–336.
19. Helgeson M J, Smith B J. Dental care in nursing homes: Guidelines for mobile and on-site care. *Spec Care Dent* 1996; **16:** 153–164.
20. Lester V, Ashley F P, Gibbons D E. Reported dental attendance and perceived barriers to care in frail and functionally dependent older adults. *Br Dent J* 1998; **184:** 285–289.
21. Office for National Statistics (99) 302; 8 Septem-

ber 1999.

22. Strayer M S. Perceived barriers to oral health care among the homebound. *Sp Care Dent* 1995; **15:** 113–118.

23. Bedi R, Devlin H, McCord J F, Schoolbread J W. Provision of domiciliary dental care for the older person by general dental practitioners in Scotland. *J Dent* 1992; **20:** 167–170.

24. Freeman R, Adams E. The prediction of dentists' work behaviour; factors affecting choice or intention in the treatment of special need patients. *Community Dent Health* 1991; **8:** 213–219.

25. Shaver D. Portable dentistry benefits homebound and providers. *N Y State Dent J* 1991; **57:** 30–31.

26. Combs R. Serving the homebound. *Dent Econ* 1994; **84:** 31–34.

27. Christensen J, Fiske J. Domiciliary Care for the Elderly Patient. In: Barnes I E, Walls A, eds. *Gerodontology*. Wright: Oxford 1994; pp.189–197.

28. Kinsey J G, Whinstanley R B. Utilisation of domiciliary dental services. *Gerodontology* 1998; **15:** 107–112.

29. Fiske J, Diu S. Undergraduate teaching in Geriatric Dentistry in the United Kingdom. *Br Dent J* 1992; **173:** 154–155.

30. British Society for Disability and Oral Health. *Development of Standards for Domiciliary Dental Care Services. Guidelines and Recommendations.* BSDH Proceedings, 1999.

Chapter 15

Integration – Implications for Oral Care

Elinor Bouvy-Berends

Introduction

In 1992 The United Nations Expert Group for Disabled defined the policy for the millennium as : 'Towards a society for all – from awareness to action.' The following objectives are aimed at people with a disability: normalisation and integration, equal opportunities and participation, de-institutionalisation and the achievement of a fully-fledged position in the community. The new paradigm is known as 'Improving Quality of Life'.

In Europe, Sweden and the other Scandinavian countries have been the forerunners in practising the principle of normalisation and integration. In the Netherlands, policies for disabled people now focus on the principle of equal opportunity. It raises the question as to whether this principle of equal opportunity can secure the same accessibility and the same standard of oral health care for disabled people, both inside and outside institutions, as for the general population. The College of Public Dental Health Officers in the Netherlands now perceive a decreasing accessibility, content and extent of oral care in the residential institutions for intellectually impaired people and psychiatric hospitals. Gabre and Gahnberg[1,2] in Sweden document a deterioration in dental health in the mildly mentally retarded population living outside the residential institutions. There is a growing 'care about oral care'. The trend to allow people with an intellectual impairment as much authority as possible over their own lives, daily activities and choices of care services, 'to act normal' has to be supported by care tailored to the individual need, together with the necessary control, to ensure 'equal opportunities' for affordable, accessible and high-quality oral health care for people with a disability as for everyone.

Consequences of 'normalisation':

- equal opportunities
- participation
- self-esteem
- autonomy
- poorer oral health

Table 1. The number of residential settings for intellectually impaired people in the Netherlands by types of facilities and their residents

Type of residential facility	Number of facilities	Residents
general institutions	90	27,170
institutions for multiply disabled	9	1,200
institutions for young intellectually impaired	19	1,900
family-replacing homes for children	20	500
family-replacing homes for adults	523	12,000
Total	661	42,700

Source: Maaskant, 1993.

Health care and welfare for disabled people in the Netherlands

The present Dutch system of care for a person with intellectual impairments is still characterised by a high degree of institutional care and need for professional resources. The risk of over-institutionalisation, however, has been recognised in recent years (*Table 1*).

In contrast, 95 per cent of all people with physical disabilities have been integrated into the existing general facilities. However, a small group in this target population is so severely disabled, often combined with cognitive deficits that they cannot use general facilities. This group unfortunately still encounters long waiting lists for specific housing and vocational facilities.

Under health care policy in the Netherlands the turning point has been reached of a movement away from 'provision based care' to a concept of care tailored to the individual's need, with integration as the basic principle[3]. The consequences of this change in policy for the oral health care planning of the disabled will be discussed (*Figure 1*).

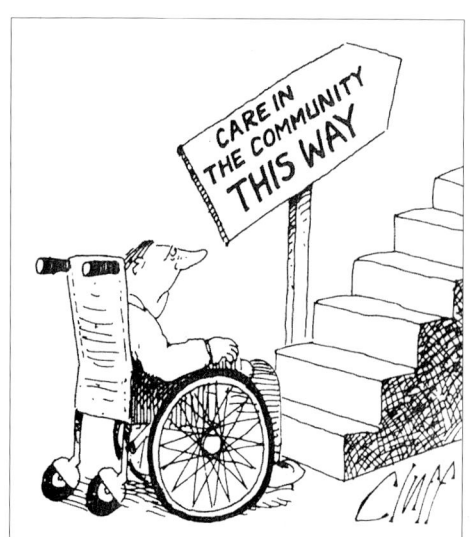

Figure 1

A cartoon from an English paper depicting the plight of people with impairments after 'normalisation' and the passing of the Care in the Community Act.

Comparison with Sweden

In Sweden and other Scandinavian countries, the principle of norma-lisation has been practised for some decades. In 1968, the construction of large-scale residential institutions in Sweden was prohibited by law. Currently, no more than 10 per cent of impaired people are institutionalised.

In 1986, the Act 'Special Services for Persons with an Intellectual Disability', was passed by the Swedish Parliament. The Act stated that the (25) counties are responsible for providing adequate care of good quality for people with an intellectual impairment. The right of self-direction of people with a disability is the central notion in this law. If the county fails to provide adequate care, the disabled individual has the right to make a legal claim. This is now the case in the United Kingdom. In this chapter it is impossible to present an extensive international comparison. Sweden is chosen because it acts, specifically for policy-makers in the Netherlands, as the role-model in the care for people with an intellectual impairment. The Swedish care system is closer to 'as normal as possible' than in most of the European countries. However, there is some concern about the availability of services in Sweden to provide special care, when needed. In 'Oral health care of the mentally retarded and other persons with disabilities in the Nordic countries. Present situation and plans for the future' Haavio[4] describes the decreasing provision of dental care for people with an intellectual impairment, due to the lack of efficient recall systems and the difficulties in dental treatment of people who are not able to co-operate in the dental chair. Gabre and Gahnberg[1,2] show the inter-relationship between the degree of intellectual impair-ment, living arrangements and dental health in adults with learning difficulties. They conclude that the degree of intellectual impairment as well as living arrangements are factors influencing the dental health of persons with this condition. A higher caries prevalence and caries incidence is seen in the mildly intellectually impaired compared to the moderate and severely impaired person. From a preventive dental health perspective, special attention should be focused on people with mild intellectual impairment, living outside institutions.

Factors resulting in a reduction of care for people with disabilities:

- lack of efficient recall systems
- challenging behaviour
- degree of intellectual impairment
- living arrangements

Trends in the care for people with an intellectual impairment

Recently the new definition by the American Association on Mental Deficiency (AAMR) [5] came into use: "Mental retardation refers to substantial limitations in present functioning. It is characterised by significantly sub-average intellectual functioning, existing concurrently with related limitations in two or more of the following applicable adaptive skill areas: communication, self-care, home living, social skills, community use, self direction, health and safety, functional academics, leisure and work. Mental retardation manifests before the age of 18".

This description implies that care for people with an intellectual impairment should be tailored to the very individual needs of this group. The ICIDH revised classification of the World Health Organisation may lead to an instrument to define a tailored approach to care [6,7].

This International Classification (IC) system distinguishes Impairments (I), disabilities (D), and (social) Handicaps (H), apart from the cause of the mental retardation. According to the International Classification of Impairment, Disability and Handicap (ICIDH), "handicap" is defined as experiencing obstacles between the person with impairments (and/or disabilities) and the existing environment. Handicaps, in this sense, are considered adaptation problems to be tackled by society, while impairments and disabilities may need individual care. By making this distinction, The ICIDH classification could be helpful in steering 'care tailored to individual needs' [8].

The objective is a valued citizenship for people with a cognitive impairment.

Oral health care for disabled people in the Netherlands: care policy and costs

The recognition of a need for a specific oral health care policy for disabled people originated mainly from the young teaching staff of the Paedodontic Department of the University of Nijmegen: Rob Burgersdijk and Willem Berendsen were the founding members of the Dutch Association of Dentistry for the Handicapped as well as the Dutch Association of Dentistry for Children, both in 1970. By that time there was a general concern by the professional organisation (Dutch Dental Association) and Health Authorities about care policy and coverage of costs for children's dentistry. A structured care service for people with a disability however had to be pursued over a longer period. Finally, in 1976 a comprehensive oral health care programme was incorporated within the coverage scheme of the Exceptional Medical Expenses Act. The alteration meant that, from then on, all institutionalised people with (severe) cognitive and physical impairments, the chronically sick and psychiatric patients could be provided with comprehensive dental care.

Oral Health Care in this context has given, from 1976 onwards, subsequent generations of dentists in the Netherlands the opportunity to provide comprehensive oral health care of good quality for patients with (severe) cognitive and physical impairments in institutions financed by the Exceptional Medical Expenses Act.

With the trend towards de-institutionalisation, a considerable number of the target population is now living in smaller residential settings where there is no longer a structured care system and coverage of costs for comprehensive oral health care. A flagrant discrepancy between facilities for oral care both inside and outside institutions has led, in 1990, to the Special Care Dentistry Regulation within the Social Health Insurance Act.

This Regulation has been designed to keep comprehensive oral health care affordable and accessible for patients with clearly defined special dental needs. This has been based on the assumption that they cannot be held responsible for their own oral health status, due to their impairment or disability. At present about 23 centres, throughout the Netherlands, can treat patients with 'special needs' (Maxillo-facial prosthetics, TMJ-dysfunction and implantology, the intellectually and physically impaired, the phobic adult and extremely anxious young child). For people with a disability, living outside institutions, this Special Care Dentistry Regulation complies with the concept of care tailored to the individual need. If the dentist can argue that a specific oral care-plan is needed in relation to the impairment or disability of the patient, costs will be fully compensated.

Oral care, according to this Special Care Dentistry Regulation can be provided as well by the general practitioner as by Centres for Special Care Dentistry. In practice, this care is mainly provided by the better skilled dentists and dental hygienists in Centres.

Legislation may be required to facilitate:

- comprehensive oral care provision
- full coverage of costs
- establishment of special care centres
- recognition of the need for care-plans

A case history

Maria, 36 years old, mildly mentally disabled with some problem behaviour, is a regular client of the Centre for Special Care Dentistry in the Rotterdam region, "BIJTER". She lives in a family-replacing or group home (GVT). In the dental office she is rather unpredictable in her changing mood; her coping abilities are restricted. She likes sweets and cannot keep her mouth clean. Inhalation sedation with nitrous oxide and oxygen is administered with varying success. The state of her oral health remains inadequate. In 1994 a session under general anaesthesia is carried out in the Centre in a day-case setting. During the peri-operative process Maria is guided by her mentor/supervisor. In 1997 the oral health status requires further treatment under general anaesthesia. The situation is different now: Maria has moved into a sheltered house (annexe of the family-replacing or group home), with less guidance and supervision. She avoids contact with her mentor and has chosen to stay regularly with her physically disabled friend Jan, who is wheelchair-bound and lives in a Fokus project home. Now we have a problem; the anaesthesiologist refuses to administer general anaesthesia as a day-case unless adequate observation of the patient at the central group home is guaranteed. But Maria is shouting to us that she will not sleep in the central home. She is furious and insists on staying the night after dental treatment in Jan's apartment. We try to calm her down by asking the full name of her boyfriend : "how would I know" she replies, and picks up her mobile telephone from her shopping bag. She enters the programmed key "1" and thus we could find out about Jan.

The end of this story?

Maria was guided during treatment by her mentor, slept that night at Jan's apartment, connected by an alarm system with the woman next door, who happens to be part of a home care organisation.

The time and energy that the Centre of Special Care Dentistry spent in this case has been out of all proportion to the care required. And let us be clear: the quality of the care process has been at risk. All went well, but only by sheer chance. We cannot be dependant on coincidences. The care process has to be handled differently.

Obviously several professionals in this case had various opinions on the ability of the client to cope independently. Although in our opinion Maria could not make a balanced decision for her own safety and dental treatment needs, her mentor allowed her this illusion by not interfering. Her lack of self care and the hindrance to apply effective preventive measures like good oral hygiene and plaque control ended inevitably in extensive dental treatment under general anaesthesia. How to find the balance between individual freedom and the responsibility of the care professionals? One could argue that in this case the wrong concept has been applied in the planning of care for this client. The lack of steering (by a mentor) in this case has put 'equal opportunity' for this patient with a cognitive impairment, at stake.

Figure 2

A letter to the British Dental Journal outlining the problems of providing adequate care for people with a disability after normalisation

Can Social Workers Damage Your Dental Health?

MADAM,—In some parts of the country, for people with a handicap it appears that the answer to this question could be yes. Since 1977 Community Dental Services have been permitted to provide dental care for handicapped adults if they could not obtain their dentistry from family dentists. More and more Community Dental Services have managed to treat people with mental handicaps who were not getting dental care previously. Some of this service involved dental screening visits at Adult Training Centres and other places, and in many health authorities a mobile dental caravan was sited at the ATC for the patients to obtain dental care. This developing service has been working reasonably well.

During the past year or two, however, social workers have been instituting a policy of 'normalisation', which means treating a person with a mental handicap as far as possible as normal. That means not treating them like children, allowing them to make their own decisions, giving them responsibility and so on.

For dentistry, in some instances, the policy of 'normalisation' has meant that social workers are denying people in the ATC a dental screening check, refusing permission for a mobile clinic to visit the centre and not accepting an offer of dental care on premises using portable dental equipment. This has resulted in many of the people with mental handicap not obtaining any dental care, as they do not in practice 'make their own arrangements with the family dentist' which is the normal thing to do. Perhaps for social workers it is normal *not* to go to dentists!

The British Society of Dentistry for the Handicapped has now obtained a written statement about this problem from the Mencap Secretary General, Sir Geoffrey Dalton, who states,

'We were concerned to hear that in implementing a policy of normalisation, Health Workers and Social Workers are, at times, refusing an offer of dental checks for people with mental handicap and not allowing help for former Residents of Long Stay Mental Handicap Hospitals to obtain a dental appointment at a specialist dental facility familiar with the needs and problems of people with mental handicap.

We find it unreasonable for a policy of normalisation to be so inflexible and inappropriate that if special facilities are needed they are denied in the name of "normalisation".

We fully support your Society in its efforts to ensure that people with mental handicap receive the dental services which they need. These views have been endorsed by our Medical Advisory Panel, and I would be most grateful if you could make them known.'

With that statement now issued, it is no longer valid for social workers to quote Mencap Policy as the reason for stopping the special dental services being provided for people with mental handicap. Let's hope that common sense will override policy where normalisation is concerned.

President,   ROBIN RIPPON.
British Society of Dentistry for the Handicapped,
Camberley,
Surrey.

Care plans

The development of a care-plan could be an instrument to bridge between professional autonomy and the freedom of the individual to make his/her own choices with regard to his medical and oral health. In an oral care-plan the dental health professionals (dentist and dental hygienist) have to decide on the objectives for oral care for the individual client/patient, taking into account his/her specific impairments and disabilities. This oral care-plan, with specific attention to preventive dental health measures has to be a part of a general care-plan. In this regard it will foster an inter-disciplinary approach to the care and welfare of people with a disability.

From present to future

Care policies for the provision of oral health care for people with disabilities is under pressure: the philosophy of empowerment of the client and the client-centred care policy requires a re-establishment of the autonomy in the process of care, of the care provider as well as the client. Undoubtedly this draws heavily on the interaction between the care-giver / care recipient. Oral health care for people with a cognitive impairment will requires a new approach: if we assign independence and responsibility to impaired people beyond their capabilities, will this lead to negligence? Conversely, if responsibility within one's limitations is denied, does this mean patronising the individual with impairments in a negative way. Where is the balance? (*Figure 2*)

The development of an oral care-plan for every client can take into account the individual need for oral health care. Consequently a dental treatment agreement can clarify the mutual responsibilities. The oral health of people with a disability, outside institutions, is at risk if responsible dental health authorities and professionals fail to adapt to the client-centred care system. Monitoring of the oral health of this potentially high risk population is paramount.

Dilemmas as a consequence of 'normalisation':

- empowerment of the person with an impairment(s)
- loss of autonomy of the care provider
- potential for dental neglect
- establishing care-plans
- professionals need to adapt to client-centred care
- lack of screening and health needs assessment

References

1. Gabre P, Gahnberg L. Dental health status of mental retarded adults with varying living arrangements. *Spec Care Dent* 1994;**14**: 203–207.
2. Gabre P, Gahnberg L. Inter-relationship among degree of mental retardation, living arrangements and dental health in adults with mental retardation. *Spec Care Dent* 1997;**17**: 7–12.
3. Magnus C. *Muren voorbij* (Beyond institutional walls).Netherlands Institute of Care and Welfare, 1993.
4. Haavio M L. Oral health care of the mentally retarded and other persons with disabilities in the Nordic countries. Present situation and plans for the future. *Spec Care Dent* 1995; **65**: 65–69.
5. Luckasson R, Coulter D L, Polloway E A, Reiss S.

Mental retardation: Definition, Classification and Systems of Supports. American Association on Mental Retardation (AAMR), Washington DC, 1992
6. World Health Organization. *International Classification of Impairments, Disabilities and Handicaps. A Manual of classification relating to the consequences of disease*. Geneva, 1980.
7. World Health Organization. *International Classification of impairments, Activities and Participation. A manual of dimensions of disablement and functioning. Beta I draft for field trials*. WHO, Geneva, 1997.
8. Ten Horn G H M M. Care for people with a Mental Handicap. In: *Health and Health Care in the Netherlands*. Schrijvers A.J.P. (ed.) Elsevier/De Tijdstroom, Maarssen, The Netherlands, 1997.

Chapter 16

Guidelines for Services

Janet Griffiths

Introduction

Disabled people are entitled to equity in health care. However within developed and industrialised societies they often experience poorer oral health and face barriers to maintaining good oral health and accessing dental services. In order to address these inequalities, it is necessary to identify:

- individuals or groups who fit agreed criteria
- patterns of health and social care provision
- normative and subjective oral health needs
- barriers to oral health
- resources to deliver appropriate oral health care and preventive measures

Services thus must focus on the needs and demands of clients, be non-discriminatory in practice and based on principles of equal access to oral health care, information and services, regardless of financial or other constraints.

Defining client groups

The concepts of impairment, disability and handicap and their potential impact on oral health are discussed in chapter 1. The individual's physical, mental or cognitive ability to carry out effective oral hygiene, seek dental services or co-operate with treatment are factors which influence oral health. Carers' ability to provide support in these activities is crucial. Early definitions of client groups largely concentrated on dental treatment and a medical model of disability, and people were described as handicapped or having 'special needs'.

'Special care' is currently the most acceptable term to disabled people in western society. The following definition of special dental care, while encompassing many earlier definitions, will be the focus for discussing guidelines for services: 'those who by virtue of illness, disease and/or its treatment, disability, life style or cultural practices, who are at greater risk of poor oral health or for whom the management of dental care poses other health risks or who experience barriers to the access and receipt of dental care'[1]. This includes physical, sensory and cognitive impairment, developmental disorders and learning disabilities, mental illness, medically compromised and emotional disability. In its widest interpretation, it includes people disadvantaged by ethnicity, social deprivation, geography or demography. People in these categories have similar oral health needs to the wider population but oral disorders impose an additional burden. They have a special need to preserve and maintain oral health, prevent pathology and obtain acceptable and accessible general and specialist dental service. There are others whose oral health needs are different from the wider population, for example the person with a craniofacial anomaly, but for whom the general principles about access to care still hold true.

Oral health needs assessment

Surveys describing oral health in people with impairments are difficult to compare due to variations in samples and methodology. However the overall picture which emerges for major disability groups is of a greater than normal unmet need for treatment, in particular, the need for significant oral hygiene input to reduce plaque and improve periodontal health.

A literature review of oral health in disabled children reports a pattern of consistently poor oral hygiene, higher levels of untreated disease and more extractions[2]. More recent studies confirm this pattern with some variation in caries experience[3–6]. Dento-facial anomalies and impaired oral function also occur with greater frequency[4,7].

A similar picture is reported for adults[5,8–12]. Oral hygiene and periodontal health is worse in institutionalised persons[12]. Disabled adults receive less dental care than non-disabled cohorts, and when treatment is provided, extractions rather than restorative care predominate[11]. Differences between sub-groups in relation to the nature and severity of disability, and residence are observed[9,11,12]. Poor oral hygiene and gingivitis are reported in paraplegics with diminished ability for self-care[13,14]. Studies report dental neglect in adults with chronic mental illness (*Figure 1*), associated with mood, motivation, lifestyle, xerostomic medication, and problems of compliance with dental attendance[15–19].

Frail or functionally dependent older people clearly fall into the category of special care. Normative need is consistently higher than subjective need both in community and residential care[20–27]. Professional concern is expressed over poor standards of oral health in residential facilities where there is evidence of considerable unmet need[20,24,27,28].

In summary, oral health profiles of people with disabilities indicate:
- greater unmet need for treatment especially amongst institutionalised populations
- more untreated caries, poorer oral hygiene, more extractions
- higher frequency of dento-facial anomalies and impaired oral function

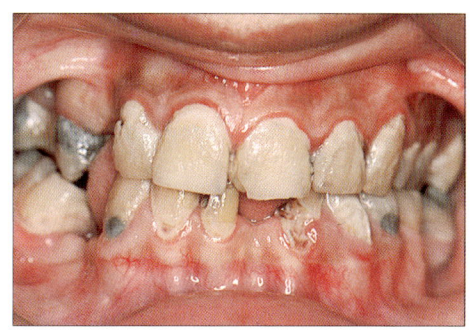

Figure 1

The neglected mouth of a patient who has a mental illness

- differences between sub-groups depending on nature and severity of impairment

Identifying target groups

An understanding of the nature of social and political systems of care and support will facilitate the identification of target groups. There are wide national, regional and local variations in health, social care and 'not for profit' support systems for care. For example in Japan, where care has largely been provided by family or philanthropic charitable organisations, legislation to support family carers has led to the development of institutionalised care systems. By contrast, in developed western societies, in accordance with the philosophy of 'normalisation', institutional care was already being replaced by 'community care' provided and supported by statutory and voluntary agencies. Integration will have an increasing impact on service development and there is concern that de-institutionalisation may result in deteriorating health, specifically oral health[29].

Collaboration with specialist services facilitates the identification of individuals who may be at risk at, or soon after, diagnosis so that ideally, a dentist would be included in the interdisciplinary team. A small proportion live in residential facilities (*Figure 2*); they can be identified with relative ease as most accommodation is registered in compliance with statutory requirements. However, since most disabled people live in their own homes (*Figure 3*), an outreach approach to health, statutory and voluntary agencies providing care and support, is a primary requirement. Networking is the key to identifying clients in the community.

Normative and subjective need

Epidemiology provides baseline data for service planning and health promotion strategies, following which screening programmes can be established. There is an ethical responsibility to advise a client of the

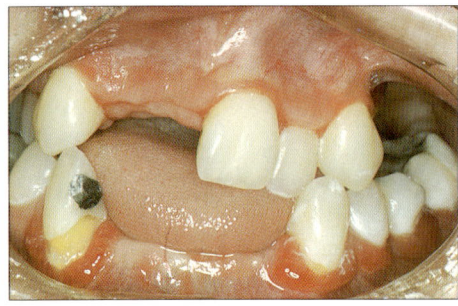

Figure 2

A woman with a learning disability in residential care whose oral state indicates a lack of comprehensive long-term treatment planning as well as an absence of adequate 'home' oral care

Figure 3

The oral state of a man with an acquired impairment – a craniopharyngioma at 15 years of age – who is reliant on his elderly mother for home oral care

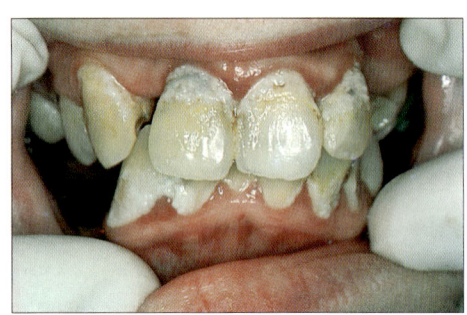

outcome of screening and ensure that resources exist to offer appropriate care. However, screening does not provide an holistic assessment of individual need and clients may decline or be unable to co-operate for examination[8,16,27].

Oral health risk assessment provides a mechanism for identifying individual needs and demands. There is no single assessment tool which weights the different factors, quantifies risk status and subsequently translates into the degree and type of intervention required.

Assessments which identify a need for referral can be adapted to different client groups[22,31]. Assessments can be self-reporting or adapted for formal and informal carers. Oral health risk assessment as part of an interdisciplinary assessment facilitates identification of a client's needs at the point of contact with professionals. This is particularly important for identifying children whose oral health is compromised by illness or disability.

The key indicators of oral health status which point towards objectives for care include:

- Presence of existing signs and symptoms of oro-dental disease
- Current mouth care practices and preventive behaviours including dental attendance patterns
- Presence of risk factors including systemic disease, medication and disability
- Presence of key stressors for oral health[30].

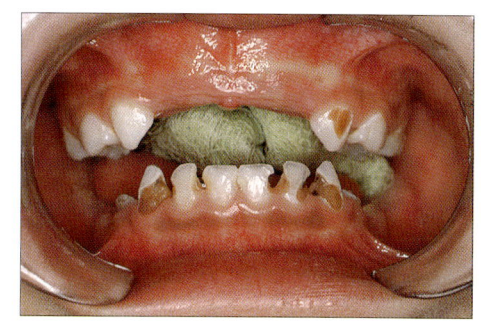

Figure 4

Delay in seeking dental care results in the extensive extraction of teeth under general anaesthesia for this child with cerebral palsy

Barriers to oral health

Disabled people form a non-homogenous group which constitute as varied and diverse a population as any group of able-bodied people. The nature and severity of disability influences the way in which an individual reacts to and copes with their situation. Service development must recognise this and address barriers, both real and perceived which individual clients experience.

Attitudes to oral health, oral hygiene, regular dental attendance, and the relative value placed on these factors must be viewed within the context of illness, disability, socio-economic status and stresses imposed upon daily living for the individual, family and/or carers. Fear and anxiety are barriers to regular dental care[16,32]. Lack of perceived need or inability to articulate need contribute to low uptake of care[18]. Those who are dependent for activities of daily living rely upon the knowledge and skill of carers for oral hygiene and access to services. Parents and carers' perception of need may reduce the frequency of contact with dental services so that treatment may be arranged only when there is a perceived problem[3,24,33]. Delays in receiving treatment lead to a greater need for extractions rather than restorative care (*Figure 4*).

Access to information, transport and physical access are consistently quoted by disabled people as being the key to independence and choice. Impaired mobility, sensory or cognitive impairment, deteriorating physical or mental health can lead to social isolation which over years conditions people to have lower expectations of services. Information needs to be widely distributed through statutory and voluntary health care and support agencies and delivered in forms which are also accessible to people with sensory impairment. It needs to be user friendly, reflect ethnic and cultural differences, presented in a way which encourages contact and reaches the target groups. Information delivery systems are largely passive and good practice dictates that at-risk groups should be specifically targeted. The quality and effectiveness of information needs to be evaluated by service users and include mechanisms to keep it up to date.

171

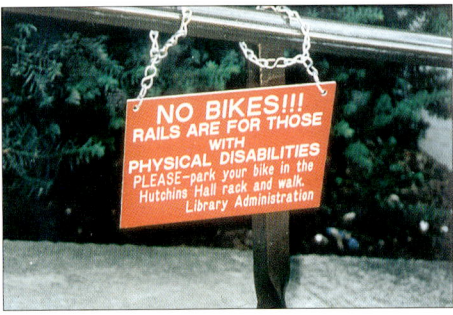

Figure 5

A sign outside the main library at the University of Michigan, Ann Arbor, USA.

The physical environment and architectural infra-structure have been constructed without reference to the needs of disabled people although anti-discrimination legislation has brought pressure for access to be a primary consideration in new buildings (*Figure 5*) Impaired mobility and ability to reach services are factors which affect the uptake of dental care[20]. Problems are caused by access to and within buildings and transport difficulties[20,34,35].

Barriers to regular dental attendance lead to delays in obtaining appropriate treatment and increase the need for crisis management for pain relief and extraction rather than preventive dental care. Oral disorders may add an additional burden for the individual who is trying to cope with their disability. Transport and physical barriers are issues which must be addressed in developing local dental services. Mobile and domiciliary services as alternative options are sometimes unacceptable within the philosophy of normalisation (see Chapter 15).

The attitudes and knowledge of health professionals and care providers are identified as barriers to oral health for those who are dependent for oral hygiene or for access to services[24,36–38]. Chronic inadequate oral hygiene practices delivered by health care workers are reported in residential facilities[24,36]. All health professionals should receive additional training to support the concept of primary oral health care[39]. However, the oral health content of professional nurse training is still reported to be inadequate[38] and few institutions support a philosophy for change in oral health care. Negotiated standards and procedures promote a structure and process for putting theory into practice and help in supporting staff in carrying out effective oral hygiene. Training for health professionals, in particular direct care providers is essential to equip them with the knowledge and skills to maintain their clients' oral health in compliance with agreed standards[28].

There is evidence of professional reluctance and unwillingness to provide dental care for disabled people[40–42]. Dentists have shown reluctance to provide care in long term care facilities, and of those providing care, few felt adequately trained[42]. Undergraduate and postgraduate training in special care dentistry is widely recommended by the International Association for Disability and Oral Health and its member organisations to redress this situation. Legislation in many countries makes it unlawful to discriminate against disabled people or treat them less favourably for a reason related to their disability[43]. This may lead to pressure for changes in professional practice. It remains to be seen whether access to dental services will be challenged under anti-discriminatory legislation.

In summary, the barriers to oral health which exist are:

Patient/carer related
- fear and anxiety
- lack of perceived need
- inability to articulate need

Professional:
- failure to recognise diversity
- failure to see oral health in the context of illness and disability
- failure to target information
- maintenance of physical and transport barriers
- inadequate staff training
- professional reluctance

Oral health care services

A range of services are necessary to satisfy the needs and demands of such a non-homogenous group: accessible general and specialist services, mobile and domiciliary care, access to out-of-hours emergency dental services and adequate resources for prompt treatment under sedation and general anaesthesia for those whose disability or anxiety limit their ability to co-operate for routine care[3,8,32]. The dental team should develop their knowledge and understanding of impairments and the way in which these disable an individual as well as their potential impact on oral health and dental management. Behaviour management, communication skills and special techniques are essential to deliver high quality care. While preventive care and treatment are a priority, there is an urgent need to reduce plaque levels and improve periodontal health by addressing the training needs of direct care providers (*Figure 6*). The role of dental auxiliaries, specifically hygienists is paramount in delivering preventive education and training.

In summary, oral health care services should be able to provide high quality:

- general and specialist oral and dental care

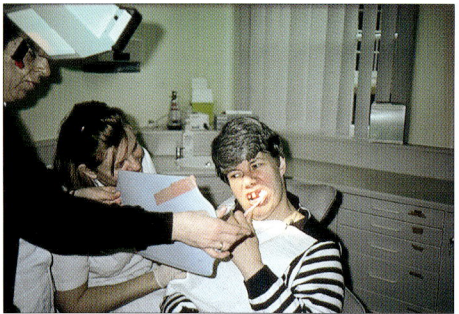

Figure 6

A hygienist demonstrates mouth cleaning techniques to a woman with a learning disability and her carer

- mobile and domiciliary care where indicated
- out-of-hours emergency care
- auxiliary help

Summary

The dental profession has a moral and ethical responsibility to reduce inequities in oral health. Clinical governance places the quality of dental care in the centre of this process. Aside from ensuring the technical excellence of clinical care, it requires services to be both accessible and appropriate. For people requiring special care, the planning and delivery of oral health care services is best achieved in partnership with disabled people and their advocates. Services should be appropriate and sensitive to individual needs, take account of the views, needs and demands of clients, family and carers, and should accord with the principles of positive choice, enhanced quality of life, retention of dignity, and wherever possible, self care. Services should specifically target populations at risk in the community and in residential care, and address the central role of carers in preservation and maintenance of oral health.

The role of oral health care services for people with impairments should:

- be responsive to needs
- take account of views and demands
- show consideration for quality of life
- respect the individual's dignity
- target high risk populations
- work in partnership with carers and other professionals

In conclusion, to quote from Clark and Vanek:'Oral health and quality oral health care contribute to holistic health. It should be a right not a privilege'[44].

References

1. Griffiths J E. *Oral health: special needs. A technical paper for the protocol for investment in health gain.* Welsh Health Planning Forum, Welsh Office, Cardiff, 1992.

2. Nunn J H. The dental health of mentally and physically handicapped children: a review of the literature. *Community Dent Health* 1987; **4**: 157–168.

3. Gizani S, Declerck D, Vinckier F, *et al*. Oral health condition of 12 year old handicapped children in Flanders (Belgium). *Community Dent Oral Epidemiol* 1997; **25**: 352–357.

4. Nunn J H, Murray J J. The dental health of handicapped children in Newcastle and Northumberland. *Br Dent J* 1987; **162**: 9–14.

5. Shapira J, Efrat J, Berkey D, *et al*. Dental health profile of a population with mental retardation in Israel. *Spec Care Dent* 1998; **18**: 149–155.

6. Vignehsa H, Soh G, Lo G L, *et al*. Dental health of disabled children in Singapore. *Aust Dent J* 1991; **36**: 151–156.

7. Storhaug K. The mentally retarded and the dental health services. Treatment needs and preventive strategies. *Nor Taanlaegeforen Tid* 1991; **101**: 262–265.

8. Francis J R, Stevenson D R, Palmer J D. Dental health and dental care requirements for young handicapped adults in Wessex. *Community Dent Health* 1991; **8**: 131–137.

9. Gabre P, Gahnberg L. Inter-relationship among degree of mental retardation, living arrangements, and dental health in adults with mental retardation. *Spec Care Dent* 1997; **17**: 7–12.

10. Kendall N P. Oral health of a group of non-institutionalised mentally handicapped adults in the UK. *Community Dental Oral Epidemiol* 1991; **19**: 357–359.

11. Shaw M J, Shaw L, Foster T D. The oral health in different groups of adults with mental handicaps attending Birmingham (UK) adult training centres. *Community Dent Health* 1990; **7**: 135–141.

12. Thornton J B, Al-Zahid S, Campbell V A, *et al*. Oral hygiene levels and periodontal disease prevalence among residents with mental retardation at various residential settings. *Spec Care Dent* 1989; **9:** 186–190.

13. Lancashire P, Janzen J, Zach G A, *et al*. The oral hygiene and gingival health of paraplegic inpatients – a cross-sectional survey. *J Clin Periodontol* 1997; **24**: 198–200.

14. Stiefel D J, Truelove E L, Persson R S, *et al*. A comparison of oral health in spinal cord injury and other disability groups. *Spec Care Dent* 1993; **13**: 229–235.

15. Angellilo I F, Nobile C G A, Pavia M, *et al*. Dental health and treatment needs in institutionalised psychiatric patients in Italy. *Community Dent Oral Epidemiol* 1995; **23**: 360–364.

16. Hede B. Oral health in Danish hospitalised psychiatric patients. *Community Dent Oral Epidemiol* 1995; **23**: 44–48.

17. Stiefel D J, Truelove E L, Menard T W, *et al*. A comparison of the oral health of persons with and without chronic mental illness in community settings. *Spec Care Dent* 1990; **10**: 6–12.

18. Whittle J G, Sarll D W, Grant A A, *et al*. The dental health of the elderly mentally ill: a preliminary report. *Br Dent J* 1987; **162**: 381–383.

19. Whyman R A, Treasure E T, Brown R H, *et al*. The oral health of long-term residents of a hospital for the intellectually handicapped and psychiatrically ill. *New Zealand Dent J* 1995; **91**: 49–56.

20. Fiske J, Gelbier S, Watson R M. Barriers to dental care in an elderly population resident in an inner city area. *J Dent* 1990; **18**: 236–242.

21. Hawkins R J. Functional status and untreated dental caries among nursing home residents aged 65 and over. *Spec Care Dent* 1999; **19**: 158–163.

22. Hoad-Reddick G. A study to determine oral health needs of institutionalised elderly patients by non dental health care workers. *Community Dent Oral Epidemiol* 1991; **19**: 233–236.

23. Lester V, Ashley F P, Gibbons D E. The relationship between socio-dental indices of handicap, felt need for dental treatment and dental state in a group of frail and functionally dependent older adults. *Community Dent Oral Epidemiol* 1998; **26**: 155–159.

24. Merelie D L, Heyman B. Dental needs of the elderly in residential care in Newcastle-upon-Tyne and the role of formal carers. *Community Dent Oral Epidemiol.* 1992; **20**: 106–111.

25. Slade G D, Locker D, Leake J L, *et al*. Differences in oral health status between institutionalised and non-institutionalised older adults. *Community Dent Oral Epidemiol* 1990; **18**: 272–276.

26. Strayer M S, Ibrahim M F. Dental treatment needs of homebound and nursing home patients. *Community Dent Oral Epidemiol* 1991; **19**: 176–177.

27. Tobias B, Smith D M. Dental screening of long stay geriatric patients in West Essex and recommendations for their care. *Community Dent Health* 1990; **7**: 93–98.

28. *Guidelines for oral care for long-stay patients and residents. Report of a working group.* British Society for Disability and Oral Health, 2000.

29. Preservation of quality oral health care services for people with developmental disabilities. A position paper from the Academy of Dentistry for Persons

with Disabilities. *Spec Care Dent* 1998; **18**: 180–182.

30. Griffiths J E, Boyle S. Oral Assessment. In *Colour Guide to Holistic Oral Care: a practical approach.* pp 87–98. Aylesbury: Mosby-Year Book Europe, 1993.

31. Griffiths J E, Williams J. Risk factors for oral health in neuro-psychiatric patients in a rehabilitation unit. *Japan Soc Dent Handicapped. Abstracts/Proceedings Supplement* 1998; **19**: 347.

32. Gordon S M, Dione R A, Snyder J. Dental fear and anxiety as a barrier to accessing oral health care among patients with special health care needs. *Spec Care Dent* 1998; **18**: 88–92.

33. deBaat C, Bruins H, Van Rossum G, *et al.* Oral health care for nursing home residents in the Netherlands – a national survey. *Community Dent Oral Epidemiol* 1993; **21**: 240–242.

34. Oliver C H, Nunn, J H. The accessibility of dental treatment to adults with physical disabilities in north east England. *Spec Care Dent* 1996; **16**: 204–209.

35. O'Donnell D. The special needs patient. Treatment in general dental practice: is it feasible? *Int Dent J* 1996; **46**: 315–319.

36. Boyle S. Assessing mouth care. *Nursing Times* 1992; **88**): 44–46.

37. Logan H L, Ettinger R, McLeran H, *et al.* Common misconceptions about oral health in the older adult: nursing practices. *Spec Care Dent* 1991; **11**: 243–247.

38. Longhurst R H. A cross-sectional study of the oral healthcare given to nurses during their basic training. *Br Dent J* 1998; **18**: 453–457.

39. Sheiham A. The Berlin Declaration on Oral Health and Oral Health Services: Berlin Declaration Summary Report. *Community Dent Health* 1993; **10**: 289–292.

40. Stiefel D J, Truelove E L, Jolly D E. The preparedness of dental professionals to treat persons with disabling conditions in long term care facilities and community settings. *Spec Care Dent* 1987; **7**: 108–113.

41. Finger S T, Jedrychowski J R. Parents perception of access to dental care for children with handicapping conditions. *Spec Care Dent* 1989; **9**: 195–199.

42. MacEntee M I, Silver J G, Gibson G, *et al.* Oral health in a long term care institution equipped with a dental service. *Community Dent Oral Epidemiol* 1985; **13**: 260–263.

43. *Disability Discrimination Act.* HMSO: London, UK, 1995.

44. Clark C A, Vanek E P. Meeting the health care needs of people with limited access to care. *J Dent Education* 1984; **48**: 213–216.